T0222213

Combatting Burnout

A Guide for Medical Students and Junior Doctors

Combatting Burnout

A Guide for Medical Students and Junior Doctors

Edited by
Adam Staten
General Practitioner
Milton Keynes, UK

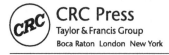

CRC Press
Taylor & Francis Group
Boca Raton London New York

CRC Press is an imprint of the
Taylor & Francis Group, an **informa** business

CRC Press
Taylor & Francis Group
6000 Broken Sound Parkway NW, Suite 300
Boca Raton, FL 33487-2742

© 2019 by Taylor & Francis Group, LLC
CRC Press is an imprint of Taylor & Francis Group, an Informa business

No claim to original U.S. Government works

Printed on acid-free paper

International Standard Book Number-13: 978-1-138-33130-3 (Paperback)
978-1-138-33136-5 (Hardback)

Library of Congress Cataloging-in-Publication Data

Names: Staten, Adam, editor.
Title: Combatting burnout : a guide for medical students and junior doctors / edited by Adam Staten.
Description: Boca Raton, FL : CRC Press/Taylor & Francis Group, [2019] | Includes bibliographical references and index.
Identifiers: LCCN 2018053382| ISBN 9781138331303 (pbk. : alk. paper) | ISBN 9781138331365 (hardback : alk. paper) | ISBN 9780429447334 (ebook)
Subjects: | MESH: Burnout, Professional--prevention & control | Medical Staff, Hospital | Students, Medical | United Kingdom
Classification: LCC R737 | NLM WA 495 | DDC 610.71/1--dc23
LC record available at https://lccn.loc.gov/2018053382

Visit the Taylor & Francis Web site at
http://www.taylorandfrancis.com

and the CRC Press Web site at
http://www.crcpress.com

Contents

Preface

The issue of occupational burnout amongst medics is not new, but it is becoming an ever bigger problem both for the individuals working within medicine but also for the whole healthcare systems within which we treat our patients. This is the first book of its kind to address the issue of burnout amongst medical students and junior doctors. By drawing on the experience and wisdom of a variety of contributors, working in different areas of medicine and at different stages of their careers, this book seeks to define the problem, explain the causes, and then offer practical solutions that can be implemented at both individual and systemic levels.

Editor

Dr Adam Staten MA MBBS MRCGP MRCP(UK) DRCOG DMCC PGCertCE, is a GP working in Milton Keynes with interests in the sustainability of the NHS and medical education. Having trained at Cambridge University and King's College London, he completed a short service commission in the Royal Army Medical Corps before returning to the NHS to complete GP training in South West London. He was also lead author and co-editor of the book *GP Wellbeing: Combatting Burnout in General Practice.*

Contributors

Ben Balogun
Emergency Medicine Trainee
United Kingdom

Ashton Barnett-Vanes
Junior Doctor
United Kingdom

Cristina Costache
Paediatric Trainee
United Kingdom

Fiona Day
Coach and Mentor
Fiona Day Consulting
United Kingdom

Mike Forsythe
GP Trainee
United Kingdom

Jonathan C. H. Lau
Junior Doctor
United Kingdom

Euan Lawson
Director of Community
Studies
Faculty of Health and
Medicine
Lancaster University

Max Marsden
Surgical Trainee
United Kingdom

Martin McShane
Former GP and Chief
Medical Officer
Optum International
United Kingdom

David N. Naumann
Surgical Trainee
United Kingdom

Lewis Potter
GP Trainee and Founder of
Geeky Medics
United Kingdom

Duncan Shrewsbury
Former Chair of the RCGP
AiT Committee
United Kingdom

Adam Staten
General Practitioner
United Kingdom

Elizabeth Waters-Dapre
Emergency Medicine Trainee
United Kingdom

Introduction

ADAM STATEN

Stress in medicine is nothing new. Stress is unavoidable in an occupation in which there is continual exposure to the suffering of others, and one in which the battle to overcome injury, sickness, and disease will always ultimately be lost. But, despite this inherent stress, and perhaps to some extent because of it, medicine is also a career that offers the opportunity for huge personal and professional satisfaction, the chance to receive respect and gratitude from those we treat, and the promise of secure, important, and potentially well-remunerated employment. It is for these reasons that a career in medicine has always attracted the brightest and the best.

However, here in the UK and elsewhere across the globe, people involved in medicine are discontent, and the level of this discontentment seems to be rising. The stresses of being a doctor are increasing as our populations grow, become older, and become more unwell, and although we can now do more than ever before for our patients, this brings with it its own extra stresses as patient expectations rise.

Today, the National Health Service (NHS) is under pressure and it is the front line staff working within it who feel this pressure most keenly. As a result, the stresses of a life in medicine are beginning to overwhelm the inherent job satisfaction of the work for many people. In recent years, we have seen industrial action from midwives and nurses and an all-out junior doctor strike for the first time in NHS history.

Across specialties, the NHS is losing doctors to early retirement, emigration, and the increasing phenomenon of doctors leaving medicine altogether. At a time when the NHS desperately needs to expand its workforce, there is instead an unprecedented recruitment and retention crisis.

At the heart of these issues is the problem of burnout. Prolonged periods of stress are psychologically unsustainable, and we are now seeing, on a large scale, doctors suffering with the mental health problems typical of the burnout syndrome. This is making large numbers of doctors less effective at their jobs, unhappy in their personal lives, and unable to continue working in the way that has become expected of them. More than this, patients are being endangered by under-filled rotas and overworked staff.

Perhaps more alarming than the level of burnout among junior doctors is the prevalence of burnout and psychological distress among medical students. It seems that those who should be the future of our profession are feeling the effects of burnout before they even take on the responsibility of caring for patients. Beyond the issue of individual suffering, from a systemic viewpoint this means that we are losing the doctors we desperately need to bolster a beleaguered work force, sometimes before they have ever worked a day in healthcare.

George Bernard Shaw said, 'the most tragic thing in the world is a sick doctor', but we are no longer talking about individual sick doctors, but a whole profession that is in need of help.

Why is this happening? Medicine still offers the opportunity for important, satisfying employment. It is a job that combines scientific learning, social skills, and organisational challenges like no other. Doctors have a more diverse array of career options than ever before and are in huge demand all over the world, with opportunities to travel, learn, research, and offer vital help to those in need in a plethora of different environments. And yet, somehow, in this world of possibilities, doctors and medical students are failing to thrive.

This book is an attempt to understand what is going on and why this is happening. More importantly, this book will seek ways to address these problems.

In doing so, we will discuss the administrative and political burdens put on doctors and the issues caused by the rising demands placed on the healthcare system by an enlarging, aging, and increasingly polymorbid population. We will also discuss the role of the media and the negative coverage that is often given to stories about health and health professionals and how this grinds down the morale of staff, and we will discuss the rising pressure of litigation and a culture of blame that is the source of so much stress. We will then explore the possible solutions to these problems, some of which will involve changing the way we work as individuals and some of which will involve changing the way that the system works.

Doctors working in a range of specialties will explain how they keep their careers fulfilling and avoid burnout by seeking out variety in their work, whether that is by undertaking business ventures, engaging in research, or finding different roles within medicine.

The nature of burnout, the nature of resilience, and what can be done to prevent one and encourage the other will be covered so that readers can better understand those things that put them at risk of burnout and those things that will protect them. As the problem of burnout becomes increasingly recognised, help is appearing, and we will also discuss where this help can be found and what can be done for those doctors or medical students who are already feeling the effects of burnout.

What I hope will be demonstrated by the end of the final chapter is that there are ways in which we can improve the way we work, improve the ways in which we approach our work, and ultimately improve the care that we provide for our patients.

1

What is burnout?

ADAM STATEN

The term burnout is used a lot and is often equated to feeling stressed by work, but burnout is more than simple stress. Burnout is a pervasive and debilitating state that results from an unsustainable period of overwhelming stress. Burnout among medical professionals is not a new phenomenon; in fact, the term was coined by the psychologist Herbert Freudenberger in 1974. Freudenberger was no stranger to stress. He was born a German Jew in Nazi Germany where his grandmother was beaten and his grandfather murdered. Still a child, he escaped on a false passport, travelling alone to New York, where he cared for himself and eventually studied for his psychology degree at night whilst working as a tool maker's apprentice by day.

But it was not these experiences that shaped his thinking on burnout. In fact, he recognised the condition in himself and colleagues whilst working in drug addiction clinics in New York, where the unrelenting emotional stress of the work had a huge psychological impact on the staff.[1]

Burnout is not limited to those working in healthcare.[2] It is a familiar concept in many areas of life, from the financial services sector to professional sports. Increasingly, burnout is recognised as a widespread issue in many walks of modern life, and this is reflected by the enormous amount of new research being conducted on the problem, not to mention the abundance of self-help literature that is published every year to help people cope with stress and burnout, whatever the cause. Burnout is, however, especially common in caring professions such as healthcare, social work, and teaching, with a prevalence of up to 25% in these professions suggested by some research.[3]

Burnout amongst doctors working within the NHS seems to be on the rise, and this is causing problems, not just for the individuals concerned, but for a healthcare system that is already desperately stretched and now at risk of losing huge numbers of staff because of it. For this reason, it is essential that we as individuals, and the system as a whole, understand what burnout is, what impact it has, and how it can be stopped or reversed.

CLINICAL FEATURES OF BURNOUT

Burnout is classically defined as an experience of physical, emotional, and mental exhaustion caused by long-term involvement with situations that are emotionally demanding.[3] It comprises three major components: emotional exhaustion, depersonalisation, and an absent sense of personal accomplishment.[4] These three major components were incorporated into a scoring system, the Maslach Burnout Inventory, which has been used to evaluate and study burnout in a variety of settings, and in a variety of guises, since its creation in 1981.[5]

When building their inventory, Maslach and colleagues defined each of these three components. They described emotional exhaustion as a feeling of being emotionally overextended by one's work. Many writers and researchers see exhaustion as the key component of the burnout syndrome, and there are alternative scoring systems to reflect this line of thought.[6,7] Exhaustion has a pervasive effect on the ability of a doctor to carry out his or her work safely and effectively or of a student to learn effectively. This feeling of exhaustion also carries over into the personal life of a burnout sufferer, affecting relationships and the ability to have a happy and fulfilling life outside of work. Thus, burnout can not only ruin careers, but it can damage all aspects of a sufferer's life, resulting in a spiral of low mood and dissatisfaction.

The second major component of burnout, depersonalisation, is described as an unfeeling, unempathetic, and impersonal response to the interaction with patients. The burnout sufferer dehumanises the person with whom they are interacting (usually the patient, although this can also be junior colleagues), and this leads to cold, callous behaviour and cynicism. The result is interactions between patient and doctor, doctor and doctor, or doctor and student that are unsatisfying, unproductive, and potentially dangerous for the patient, as well as potentially damaging to the doctor's career. This type of interaction also contributes to a diminished sense of personal accomplishment for the doctor, which is the third component of the burnout syndrome.

Personal accomplishment relates to a sense of competence or achievement in one's work which results in job satisfaction or, if absent, dissatisfaction. A poor sense of personal accomplishment has been demonstrated by some studies to be the leading feature of burnout amongst certain groups of medical professionals such as physicians working in pain management in the US.[8]

The Maslach Burnout Inventory uses a questionnaire from which a score can be given to each of these three features to identify those who are suffering from burnout and those who are at risk of burnout. This sterile, statistical way of considering a human problem is particularly useful for research, but the real-life interaction between these three components varies considerably, resulting in different degrees of distress and debilitation for sufferers.

There are a number of factors that can contribute to occupational burnout, whatever the occupational environment. In general, people are at high risk of occupational burnout when they do not feel in control of their work. Workload can be an issue, but it is actually the ability to manage that workload by being able to make decisions and take control of the way it is managed that is key. In the literature, the ability to make these crucial decisions is known as decision latitude. If you lack decision latitude with regards to workload management, then this can lead to unsustainable workplace stress and burnout.[9]

It is easy to see how junior doctors and medical students can be robbed of decision latitude, being, as they are, at the whim of rota coordination, patient flow, and service demand. Related to a lack of decision latitude are dysfunctional workplace dynamics (i.e. management and senior colleagues preventing juniors making these decisions), which may also include workplace bullying and an unclear or ill-defined job role.

Burnout can be the result of work that is monotonous or work that is chaotic, or indeed work that combines elements of these two apparently conflicting features.[4] Work within healthcare is often capable of combining these two elements, with mundane routine work frequently interspersed with complex, important, and emotionally demanding tasks. Perhaps this is why those working within healthcare find themselves at such high risk of burnout.

Low income can also be a factor, as demonstrated in a study of burnout among paediatric nurses.[10] Like the paediatric nurses in the study, junior doctors working at the bottom end of the pay scale may feel themselves under-rewarded for the work they do and, of course, medical students have not yet even made it onto the pay scale. A poor work–life balance is another contributing factor to burnout and one that is not limited to healthcare professionals.[2]

Some people are naturally predisposed to burnout due to their nature. Unfortunately the personality traits most linked to burnout, which include perfectionism, competitiveness, and the need to feel in control, along with habitual high achievement, are traits that are often actively sought by medical schools. We therefore take people who are by nature at risk of burning out and put them into an environment where a degree of burnout is all but inevitable.

IMPACT ON THE INDIVIDUAL

There is a big overlap between the symptoms of burnout and those of anxiety and depression with all three conditions having both psychological and physical symptoms. Typically burnout is thought to progress through three stages, each with a characteristic suite of symptoms.[11]

The first stage of the burnout syndrome is known as stress arousal and is typified by difficulty concentrating, memory lapses, irritability, and anxiety. Physical symptoms, like those associated with anxiety disorders, include teeth grinding, palpitations, headaches, poor sleep, and loss of libido.

The second stage is the period of energy conservation during which people begin trying to find ways to compensate for the stress they are under. We all have ways of coping with stress, but it is at this point that a burnout sufferer's usual ways of coping are overwhelmed. This can result in maladaptive coping strategies which often exacerbate the problem in the long run.

These maladaptive strategies include avoidance behaviours such as lateness, procrastination, social withdrawal, and increased, unscheduled time off work through sick leave. Avoidance may also be manifested by difficulty with decision making and problem solving, which, as might be imagined, presents a real problem for the occupational functioning of a doctor (Figure 1.1).

It is during this period that exhaustion can set in and psychological problems increase possibly leading to self-medication with drugs or alcohol, another maladaptive coping strategy that can also cause deterioration in occupational functioning.

The third and final stage of burnout is exhaustion. This stage is associated with chronic mental health problems such as anxiety and depression, and even suicidality. People at this stage of burnout may increasingly rely on substance misuse as a coping strategy, so addiction may be a concurrent problem. Feelings of apathy are common and decision making is poor, leading to poor patient care and unethical behaviour.[11] Somatic symptoms which may also be present include non-cardiac chest pain, dizziness, and chronic headaches.

There need not be an inexorable progression through these three stages. If we are able to recognise these symptoms, either in ourselves or in our colleagues, then appropriate measures can be put in place to halt and reverse the onset of burnout.

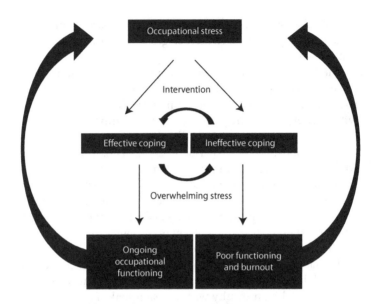

Figure 1.1 The cycle of stress and burnout.

However, if the problem is not recognised and is left untended, the long term consequences, both physical and mental, can be severe. Physical health problems that have been linked to occupational stress include an increased rate of myocardial infarction, and a poor prognosis following an ischaemic event, the metabolic syndrome, and even a postulated link with the formation of stones in the urinary tract.[12-14] Burnout is very bad for your health.

Substance misuse and addiction are also strongly associated with occupational burnout. Between 10% and 15% of US physicians are thought to suffer with a substance misuse disorder. In 1998, a British Medical Association (BMA) working group found that around one in 15 doctors in the UK had some form of dependence on alcohol or drugs, and it is thought that, in the decades since, that drug and alcohol misuse has increased with the availability of novel psychoactive substances and a permissive social attitude to binge drinking.[15,16] This can have a huge impact on professional and social functioning, and it is often a problem that is compounded by the reluctance of doctors to seek help. There is also evidence that burnout can result in the development of eating disorders, including overeating, leading to the individual becoming overweight or obese.[17]

This wide range of physical and psychological symptoms results in doctors ceasing to work effectively within the NHS, or otherwise recognising that there is a problem and leaving work within the NHS entirely. This has knock-on effects for the wider NHS workforce, who must then take up the slack which puts them under more stress.

EFFECT ON THE NHS WORKFORCE

Junior doctors comprise an enormous part of the NHS workforce, providing huge amounts of the care, treatment, and decision making in the health system. It used to be taken for granted that doctors in the UK would generally stay within the NHS from the day they qualified until the day they retired.

This is no longer the case, and for all the reasons that junior doctors are burning out (to be discussed in later chapters), they are also seeking the solutions of leaving the NHS, leaving the country, or leaving medicine altogether.

Rota gaps are almost universal, with the National Audit Office estimating that the NHS was short of 2550 doctors in 2017, a situation that has been steadily deteriorating.[18] Some specialties are feeling the pinch more than others, for example 20% of paediatric training posts were unfilled in 2017, and in the same year, the Royal College of Physicians found that 84% of its members were struggling to properly staff rotas, and this was leading to concern about patient safety.[19,20]

This situation is hardly surprising given the steady decline in the number of doctors progressing into specialty training following their foundation programme. This figure fell year on year between 2011 and 2015 from 75% to just 52%,[21] which poses not just an immediate concern about staffing rotas now, but a real problem for those involved with future workforce planning who are simply not seeing the expected number of consultants emerging after the expected time period for any given cohort of new doctors.

BURNOUT: MY EXPERIENCE

Dr Mike Forsythe, GP Trainee

'Are you okay? Do you need to take a few minutes?'

I looked up, the large brown eyes of Janette barely inches from my own. There was concern etched upon her face. More concern, it occurred to me, than I could muster for anyone else at that moment, or at any moment over the previous week.

We were in the store cupboard, ostensibly because it was the first place I could think of that would be away from prying eyes elsewhere in the emergency department, but in reality it was because I'd just stormed out of a patient's cubicle, halfway through a consultation.

I'd had to do it. I'd had to turn around and just walk out midway through the conversation. It was rude, and it was definitely unprofessional, but the alternative was much worse; I was going to swear at the patient. I was going to say something I'd regret, and something I could never take back.

There wasn't even anything particularly memorable about this particular patient. He was angry that he wasn't getting what he wanted, and he was aggressive, but he wasn't the first who'd arrived in the emergency department expecting an MRI at 10 p.m., and he certainly wouldn't be the last to demonstrate dissatisfaction by raising his voice and pointing a finger in my face. Instead, he was the straw, as they say, that broke the camel's back. He was the culmination of a brutal week in an emergency department, a chaotic sleep pattern, and a non-existent social life.

The emergency department rota had broken me. I'd worked four of the previous five weekends and more night shifts than I could remember. The staffing was skeletal.

Most of the registrars were locums. The consultant of the day would greet us at the start of every shift with an expression of either panic or resignation.

I forced myself to smile at Janette. She has kind and she genuinely cared, but she was busy, so I told her I was okay. It was a lie though, because something had changed.

Later that evening I stared at my reflection in the mirror, barely recognising the figure looking back at me. I was thinner, and I had acne for the first time in years. Worse still, an eczematous rash had broken out over my face and neck. It could be stress, the GP had told me, and it was hard to disagree.

I'd not planned on moving back to Australia. I'd worked there already after my foundation years, and returned to the UK with the intention of dedicating myself to a career in the NHS. This is where I'd trained, and like many doctors working in the UK, I was fiercely loyal to the concept of the health service. I was aware how difficult it could be, I accepted the unique challenges that the NHS provided, and I was ready for it.

I wasn't prepared, though, to feel like this. All that loyalty, that drive, had disappeared, because all of it – the patient, the hospital, the system – had become the enemy. I was exhausted, demoralised, and one more bad shift away from tearing up my medical degree and leaving the profession for good. When the opportunity presented itself, then, to go back to Australia and leave the NHS behind, it was an easy decision.

The prospect of a change saw me through the final few months, and before long, I was on the other side of the world. I was working in an emergency department again, and although the job was still stressful, the workload was lighter and the rota more manageable. The change itself had done some good too, and after a few months, I felt back to normal. The rash had faded, my enthusiasm had returned, and I no longer dreaded the prospect of work.

EFFECT ON THE NHS

The effect of losing doctors and under-filled rotas is clearly a big and current problem for the whole NHS. Accident & Emergency waiting times are the usual barometer by which the pressure on the NHS is measured, and it is clear from the steadily increasing waiting times and the declining number of patients being seen within four hours, that there is a problem (Figure 1.2).

Plugging the rota gaps caused by this shortage of doctors is also of financial cost to NHS trusts who are forced to fill them with locums, and locums are now operating in a sellers' market, with desperate acute trusts bidding against one another to secure doctors on a shift-by-shift basis. Medical locums cost the NHS over £1 billion per year and, this, despite concerted efforts to reduce the reliance on temporary staff and changes to tax laws that were intended to make it less appealing to work as a locum.[22]

These immediate problems of staffing and finances cannot simply be seen through the narrow lens of today. The loss of junior doctors to the system may pose an existential threat to the NHS not least because, whilst financial problems could be rectified swiftly if there was a political will to do so, training a new workforce will take many years.[23]

Moreover, there is a push for doctors to take up more leadership positions within the NHS, and it has been speculated that a cohort of increasingly burnt-out and jaded doctors taking up leadership and management positions may be extremely damaging for the future structure and functioning of the NHS.[24]

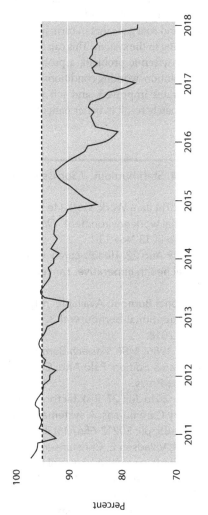

Figure 1.2 Performance against the emergency department four-hour standard. (Adapted from Performance against the A&E four-hour standard: type 1 and type 3 units in 'How is the NHS performing?' March 2018 quarterly monitoring report', Murray et al., The King's Fund (report), 8 March 2018 (https://www.kingsfund. org.uk/publications/how-nhs-performing-march-2018). Reproduced with permission.)

CONCLUSION

The spectre of burnout is a problem at individual, specialty, and whole-system levels. In the NHS, doctors are at risk of being trapped in a vicious circle of staff shortage and rota gaps that in turn, intensify the stress put upon those left working in the system. This can be changed. If burnout is recognised as a systemic problem, a problem which therefore requires a systemic solution, working conditions for doctors can be improved, retention rates improved, and job satisfaction increased, and this would ultimately result in better patient care.

REFERENCES

1. Freudenberger HJ. 1974. Staff burnout. *J Soc Issues*. 30(1): 159–165.
2. Hammig O, Bauer GF. 2014 Jan. Work, work-life conflict and health in an industrial work environment. *Occup Med (Lond)*. 64(1): 34–8, Epub 2013 Nov 13.
3. Mateen FJ, Dorji C. 2009 Aug 22. Health-care worker burnout and the mental health imperative. *Lancet*. 374(9690): 595–597.
4. Tidy C. 2015. Occupational Burnout. Available: http://patient.info/doctor/occupational-burnout#ref-3. Accessed: 19th August 2018.
5. Maslach C, Jackson SE. 1986. *MBI: Maslach Burnout Inventory; Manual Research Edition*. Palo Alto, CA: Consulting Psychologists Press.
6. Gómez-Urquiza JL et al. 2016 Jun 27. Risk factors and burnout levels in Primary Care nurses: A systematic review. *Aten Primaria*. 49(2): 77–85, pii: S0212-6567(16)30175-5.
7. Kristensen TS, Borritz M, Villadsen E, Christensen KB. 2005. The Copenhagen burnout inventory: A new tool for the assessment of burnout. *Work and Stress*. 19(3): 192–207.
8. Kroll HR, Macaulay T, Jesse M. 2016 Jul. A preliminary survey examining predictors of burnout in pain medicine physicians in the United States. *Pain Physician*. 19(5): E689–96.

9. Wong CA, Spence Laschinger HK. 2015 Dec. The influence of frontline manager job strain on burnout, commitment and turnover intention: A cross-sectional study. *Int J Nurs Stud*. 52(12): 1824–33.

10. Akman O, Ozturk C, Bektas M, Ayar D, Armstrong MA. 2016 Jun 7. Job satisfaction and burnout among paediatric nurses. *J Nurs Manag*. 24(7): 923–933.

11. School of Greenville Medicine. 2013. Medical Student Stress and Burnout. Available: http://greenvillemed. sc.edu/doc/Medical%20Student%20Stress%20and%20 Burnout%20Feb%202013.pdf. Accessed: 19th August 2018.

12. Consoli SM. 2015 Jul–Aug. Occupational stress and myocardial infarction. *Presse Med*. 44(7–8): 745–51.

13. Almadi T, Cathers I, Chow CM. 2013 Sep. Associations among work-related stress, cortisol, inflammation, and metabolic syndrome. *Psychophysiology*. 50(9): 821–830.

14. Arzoz-Fabregas M et al. 2013 Apr. Chronic stress and calcium oxalate stone disease: is it a potential recurrence risk factor? *Urolithiasis*. 41(2): 119–127.

15. Oreskovich MR et al. 2012. Prevalence of alcohol use disorders among American surgeons. *Arch Surg*. 147: 168–174.

16. Royal College of Psychiatrists. 2011. Pychiatrists' support service: On Drug and Alcohol Problems. Available: https://www.rcpsych.ac.uk. Accessed: 19th August 2018.

17. Nevanpera NJ et al. 2012 Apr. Occupational burnout, eating behavior, and weight among working women. *Am J Clin Nutr*. 95(4): 934–43.

18. National Audit Office. 2016. Managing the supply of NHS clinical staff in England. Report by the Comptroller and Auditor General HC 736.

19. Royal College of Paediatrics and Child Health. 2017. Rota compliance and vacancies. The Royal College of Paediatrics and Child Health.

20. Royal College of Physicians. 2017. Physicians worried about future patient safety, whistleblowing and rota gaps. Royal College of Physicians.

21. BMJ Careers 8/2/17, 'Half of doctors don't go straight into specialty training'.
22. NHS Improvement. 2017. Agency controls: £1 billion saving and new measures.
23. Nuffield Trust. 2017. The NHS workforce in numbers: Facts on staffing and staff shortages in England. Available: www.nuffieldtrust.org.uk/resource/the-nhs-workforce-in-numbers. Accessed: 19th August 2018.
24. Imo U. 2017 Aug. Burnout and psychiatric morbidity among doctors in the UK: A systematic literature review of prevalence and associated factors. *BJPsych Bull.* 41(4): 197–204.

2

Pressures of the job

MIKE FORSYTHE

Ever since the threat of industrial action became a reality in early 2016,[1] the life of the junior doctor, and the nature of the job they perform, has captured the public imagination.

There have been attempts in the media to portray junior doctors as champagne-swilling reprobates, but for the most part there has been support and a new-found understanding of the pressures of working in the NHS.[2] Graduates from medical school can be as young as twenty-two years old, thrust into roles in which decisions can impact upon life and death. Combined with the pressures that affect new employees in any job – getting to grips with an unfamiliar working environment and the expectations of seniors, for instance – the start of a career in medicine can be particularly daunting.

The rates of burnout and mental illness in junior doctors are high. The reasons for this are complex and no doubt multifactorial, but with as many as 60%[3] of a profession focused on the wellbeing and care of others found to be experiencing their own health issues, there are bound to be serious concerns about the retention of the workforce within the NHS.

The prevalence of burnout in Australian doctors was addressed in 2008 by the Australian Medical Association via a survey on the health and wellbeing of junior doctors. The results they obtained suggested that 69% of the respondents were at risk of burnout (73% of females and 65% of males).[4] The study also suggested that 54% of the respondents were at risk of compassion fatigue, defined as 'the stress resulting from wanting to help a traumatised or suffering person'.[5] Furthermore, 71% of the respondents had lower than average levels of job satisfaction, which is a key feature of the burnout syndrome.

A study performed in the UK showed similar results, with burnout scores for emotional exhaustion ranging from 31% to 54.3%.[6] Factors cited as contributing towards burnout were job dissatisfaction, increase in workload, and having to work longer hours. Once present, there seems to be a high chance of burnout persisting, with a US study showing that 72% of medical residents found to be suffering with burnout symptoms continued to have persistent symptoms throughout their three years of training.[7]

The job of being a junior doctor has always been stressful, but why is it that junior doctors are experiencing such high levels of burnout today? This chapter will explore the factors inherent in the job of a junior doctor that predispose junior doctors to burnout.

CHANGING PRESSURES OF WORKLOAD

The NHS as a whole is experiencing pressures like never before.[8] Faced with an ageing population, an increase in demand for social care,[9] and dwindling staffing numbers in certain specialties, the future of the healthcare system as we know it appears uncertain. Junior doctors, in their role on the frontline, are bound to feel the effect of this as keenly as any.

The NHS deals with approximately one million patients every 36 hours, and the demand on the service has increased exponentially over the last decade. In the year 2015–2016, there were 40% more operations carried out, 28% more hospital admissions, and 23.5% more attendances to A&E than in 2005–2006.[10]

Not only have patient numbers increased, but the cases are now more complex than ever before, with patients frequently presenting with multiple long-term conditions, either as a complicating factor of an acute admission or as a direct cause for that admission. In 2018, the number of patients being classed as having more than one long-term condition rose to 2.9 million, which is 1 million more complex patients than were living a decade earlier.[11] Without a comparative increase in medical staff, and in the provision of medical services, there are going to be problems dealing with this skyrocketing demand on the health service which will inevitably impact on those working within it.

ROTA GAPS

There are fewer candidates applying to medical school than ever, and given the persistently pessimistic coverage of the NHS in the media, it is easy to understand why this may be the case. Applications to foundation training are also decreasing, as are the number of training positions available. Many doctors are now taking time out after their foundation years, and in 2016, almost three quarters of specialty training programmes faced under-recruitment. The knock-on effect of this is problems with staffing, and more pertinently, gaps in the junior doctor rota.[12]

Work ordinarily carried out by two doctors is now being managed by one. It is a daily experience for many to find that their colleagues are suddenly unfamiliar locums who often need help with access to information technology (IT), or familiarization with local protocols and pathways, and who have varying degrees of experience and competence.

Staffing of medical teams is often skeletal, with no spare capacity to cope with sickness or fluctuating workload intensity. Because of this, doctors regularly find themselves working beyond their contractual hours, whether due to concerns about patient safety, or simply because there is no one else available to cover their role. In a recent UK-wide General Medical Council (GMC) survey, over half admitted to working beyond their rostered hours, and one in four had experienced difficulty sleeping as a result of their job.[13]

These problems with staffing impact upon educational opportunities, too. Where the first two years post graduation are supposed to be an opportunity for new doctors to find their feet and benefit from first-hand teaching and supervision, increasingly their time is entirely occupied with service provision; there are fewer of the learning opportunities that provide moments of interest and the potential for increased job satisfaction that are important both for professional development and for avoiding burnout. Rather than being afforded educational opportunities on the wards or in clinics, junior doctors are instead finding themselves isolated, unsupervised, and desperately trying to keep their heads above water.

Perhaps perversely, the legislation that was intended to limit the excesses of working hours, the European Working Time Directive, has actually increased the stress of work for many junior doctors. With doctors working fewer hours across the week, hospitals have been forced to move to shift-based rotas, and this has led to the breakdown of the traditional firm structure of hospital medicine. Whereas junior doctors had previously worked in tight-knit teams that worked together from the point of admitting patients to the point of their discharge, a shift system means that doctors who nominally work in the same team or specialty may seldom cross paths as they are pulled away for on-calls, night shifts, and rest days. This results in a more lonely way of working and, whilst the number of hours worked has become more manageable, those hours are often spent feeling isolated and unsupported.

PATIENT EXPECTATIONS

There has been a shift in the dynamics of the doctor–patient relationship. Gone are the days of paternalistic care and the word of a doctor being deemed as gospel. Instead the decision processes in medicine today are far more two-sided, with patient-centred care putting the needs of the patient front and centre in every consultation. This is undoubtedly a better and more ethical approach to the practice of medicine, but it comes with greater expectations on the part of patients and a greater responsibility on the part of doctors to explain and justify their decisions.

Many patients arrive with a particular agenda, which may be fed by information from social media or the internet, and they may leave unhappy and resentful if this agenda isn't met, especially if the reasons why it has not been met are not clearly explained. In the age of instant gratification, and a multitude of non-healthcare based services available at the mere touch of a button, patients will often not tolerate delays in their management.

Patients today are far more informed about their symptoms, illnesses, and potential treatments than ever before. Managing expectations can be difficult, time-consuming, and often frustrating. Demand inevitably outstrips supply in a resource-strapped system. There are often waiting lists, or limitations on the care doctors can offer. Failing to give the care that patients often quite reasonably expect, and managing the conflicts that can ensue because of this, is a burden for medical staff.

Every doctor wants the best for their patients, and it can be easy to feel guilty if the care you provide leads to disappointment or discontent. This, in turn, can lead to a breakdown in the doctor-patient relationship or, even worse, complaints and litigation. In a GMC survey, a rise in patient expectations was cited as one of the reasons for a 100% rise in complaints between the years of 2007 and 2012.[14]

EMOTIONAL IMPACT

The emotional repercussions of dealing with the sick and the dying can be substantial. Despite the traditional teaching of 'detached concern', most people entering the medical profession are by nature empathic, and many would consider the emotional element of the job one of its most rewarding features.

Unfortunately, the relentless nature of the job gives little time to debrief or reflect on a difficult clinical encounter before there is another patient to be seen or another job to be completed.

Compassion fatigue, and ultimately, the depersonalization typical of burnout, is all too common as a result.

A study carried out in 2007 attempted to investigate the impact that patient deaths had upon the doctors involved. It demonstrated that between 5% and 17.5% of doctors experienced emotional reactions classified as moderate to severe in response to a memorable recent patient death. The study suggests that, although most doctors consider that they deal well with patient death, many of us are strongly affected by patient deaths regardless of experience, specialty, or gender.[15] This then begs the question of how we prepare ourselves for these experiences and how we support each other through them when they occur, topics that will be discussed in later chapters.

Another study from 2017 showed that the prevalence of psychiatric morbidity ranged from 17% to 52% in junior doctors in the UK.[6] Doctors fear the repercussions of being branded 'mentally ill' and often seek help late, or not at all as a result, as demonstrated by a study from 2011 which showed that around 74% would disclose problems to a friend or family member rather than a professional, citing possible career implications as their reason for doing so.[16] Doctors can therefore experience a toxic combination of severe emotional distress and a reluctance to get the help they need.

CONCLUSION

Both anecdotal reports and formal studies into burnout suggest that the rate of burnout amongst junior doctors is worryingly high. There are numerous factors that might be contributing towards this, but certainly the rising pressures associated with working as a doctor in the NHS, along with the reticence from juniors themselves to admit if there is a problem, are two important issues to consider.

Senior doctors and others responsible for the training of juniors and students must begin to acknowledge that there is an issue with burnout; the 'in *my* day' attitude of demeaning the workloads of juniors nowadays compared to years gone by is disingenuous and is potentially increasing the reluctance of those who need help to ask for it.

REFERENCES

1. http://www.independent.co.uk/news/uk/home-news/junior-doctors-strike-contract-dispute-timelines-bma-jeremy-hunt-nhs-a7001061.html

2. Mori I. 25th April 2016. Majority Support Junior Doctors Ahead of First Full Walkout. Available: www.ipsos.com/ipsos-mori/en-uk/majority-support-junior-doctors-ahead-first-full-walkout. Accessed: 19th August 2018.

3. Cohen D, Winstanley SJ, Greene G. 1 July 2016. Understanding doctors' attitudes towards self-disclosure of mental ill health. *Occup Med.* 66(5): 383–389.

4. Australian Medical Association. 2008. AMA survey report on junior doctors health and wellbeing. Available: https://ama.com.au/article/ama-survey-report-junior-doctor-health-and-wellbeing. Accessed: 19th August 2018.

5. Figley C (ed) 1995. *Compassion Fatigue: Coping with Secondary Traumatic Stress in Those Who Treat the Traumatised.* New York: Brunner/Mazel.

6. Imo UO. 2017 Aug. Burnout and psychiatric morbidity among doctors in the UK: A systematic literature review of prevalence and associated factors. *BJPsych Bull.* 41(4): 197–204.

7. Campbell J, Prochazka AV, Yamashita T, Gopal R. 2010 Oct. Predictors of persistent burnout in internal medicine residents: A prospective cohort study. *Acad Med.* 85(10): 1630–4.

8. NHS England. 2017. Five Year Forward View: Next Steps. Available: www.england.nhs.uk/five-year-forward-view/next-steps-on-the-nhs-five-year-forward-view/the-nhs-in-2017/#one. Accessed: 19th August 2018.

9. King's Fund. 2017. Priorities for NHS and Social Care in 2017. Available: https://www.kingsfund.org.uk/publications/priorities-nhs-social-care-2017. Accessed: 19th August 2018.

10. NHS Confederation. 2017. Key Statistics on the NHS. Available: http://www.nhsconfed.org/resources/key-statistics-on-the-nhs. Accessed: 19th August 2018.

11. Department of Health. 2012. *Long-Term Conditions Compendium of information*. 3rd ed.
12. British Medical Association. September 2017. The state of pre and post-graduate medical recruitment in England.
13. British Medical Association. 2017. Training Survey Exposes Rota Gap Dangers. Available: https://www.bma.org.uk/news/2017/july/training-survey-exposes-rota-gap-dangers. Accessed: 19th August 2018.
14. General Medical Council. 2014. What's Behind the Rise in Complaints About Doctors from Members of the Public? Available: https://gmcuk.wordpress.com/2014/07/21/whats-behind-the-rise-in-complaints-about-doctors-from-members-of-the-public/. Accessed: 19th August 2018.
15. Moores TS, Castle KL, Shaw KL, Stockton MR, Bennett MI. 2007 Oct. 'Memorable patient deaths': Reactions of hospital doctors and their need for support. *Med Educ.* 41(10): 942–6.
16. Brooks SC, Gerada C, Chalder T. 2011. Review of literature on the mental health of doctors: Are specialist services needed? *J Ment Health*. 20: 1–11, iFirst article.

3

External pressures

CRISTINA COSTACHE AND ADAM STATEN

Interactions between doctor and patient can be immensely satisfying and, in some ways, if our jobs just involved the work of seeing our patients, life would be very much simpler. However, we cannot work in isolation. We work within complex healthcare systems that have to deliver care to entire populations, and we are accountable not only to our patients, but also to our colleagues, our government, and, particularly in the case of the NHS, to the tax-paying public at large.

Where do you fall in all this as a junior doctor? When it comes to our training and our service provision, we all carry a heavy burden of expectations, both from ourselves and others: never to be ill, never to be tired, and to work always at our full potential.

Whole institutions, such as the GMC, Royal Colleges, or the care quality commission (CQC), exist to ensure that we do the job we are supposed to do. Evidencing that we are trained to the required level and that we are working in a satisfactory way brings with it an enormous burden of stress, in addition to those stressors inherent to the work of caring for our patients.

MILESTONES IN OUR CAREER

While you are being asked to give your all at work, you need a special pocket full of energy specially kept for exams. Exams are expensive and time consuming – they involve doing questions on the train or bus, while walking on the street, before bed, and while eating breakfast. Revising for exams can make you feel like you are back at medical school, but at medical school, studying was a full-time occupation; as a junior doctor, it is a burden added on top of a full-time job. Unfortunately, they are a necessary evil if you are to advance in your career. Achieving membership to a Royal College can also cost thousands of pounds, even assuming you sail through each exam first time.

Whilst sitting (and passing) membership exams can be rewarding and satisfying, the same is rarely said of the treadmill of the Annual Review of Competence Progression (ARCP). This annual tick-box exercise is another necessary evil to climb the ladder to consultancy. From reflections to case-based discussions and meetings, quality improvement projects, and audits, the work involved in getting all the right boxes ticked can be time consuming and stressful, particularly when senior colleagues are difficult to pin down for the crucial assessments. Again, these are things to be completed in addition to providing a healthcare service to our patients. This tick-box approach to career progression was cited by many junior doctors in a report for the Royal College of Physicians as a major source of dissatisfaction, with many feeling that it actually detracted from having meaningful educational conversations with their seniors.[1]

Despite all this endeavour to climb the career ladder, what is a modern career actually like and how do we make decisions about our career path? Spooner et al. studied how and why junior doctors make career decisions in the UK and found how important a good work–life balance is for doctors when it comes to choosing their career path.[2] This meant not only the time for their family and friends (i.e. life outside of medicine), but also the variety of life inside of medicine and outside the borders of their own specialty. Between 1996 and 2012, they examined patterns in the amount of leisure time that junior doctors get. Although they found that junior doctors now work fewer hours, this was counterbalanced by an increase in workload and an increase in less sociable hours. This suggests that, whilst overall hours worked are less, the working hours may be more intense and are being worked at more unsociable times such as nights and weekends. These unsociable hours are compensated for by time off during the week, but these extra hours gained outside of work are not necessarily useful for leading a satisfying personal life.

The same study also found the detrimental effect of the loss of a traditional medical team and the resultant loss of camaraderie, support, and continuity of care for patients – elements that used to have a significant positive impact on a junior doctor's working life.[2] Bleakly, this study suggests that junior doctors are making career choices simply to mitigate the effects of working in an increasingly intense and lonely environment.

These findings were reflected more recently in the GMC's 2016 national training survey, which highlighted the effect that the workload had on training: 43% of junior doctors responded that their daytime workload was 'heavy' or 'very heavy', 2.3% more than in 2012, and the doctors in this group had twice as many concerns about patient safety in their post compared with doctors who said that their workload was about right. Under such pressures, how could the quality of work not to be affected?[3] This concern about patient safety then feeds into concerns about complaints and litigation, an added source of stress for doctors (discussed below).

In 'Being a junior doctor: Experiences from the front line of the NHS', published by the Royal College of Physicians in 2016, 41% of junior doctors reported feeling that the burden of their administrative work actually posed a threat to the safety of their patients.[1]

WE ARE HUMAN

As much as it seems that we spend our entire time in the hospital, we actually don't. We are all human, we do wish to have a family and to keep contact with friends, however we have to battle with quite an antisocial program. We miss birthdays, anniversaries, weddings, school plays, and good-night stories. The collision between the passion for your profession and for the ones that care for you is difficult to manage. The NHS, and the work that it needs us to perform, stops for nothing, even illness. Illness, whether it's the illness of your child, your parents, or even yourself, is frequently seen as a disaster in our over-stretched NHS teams who have to pick up the slack if you aren't there to work.

It is difficult to escape the feeling that while you're at work wishing for your set of nights to end, your parents are growing older, your children are learning new words and discovering the world without you, and your friends are making memories in which you will never be remembered.

Maintaining a connection with friends and family is also hindered by the frequent moves both within a region and between regions at every stage in our career. Moves within a region can occur every few months, but moves to new jobs may be to completely new parts of the country with every major change in career stage – after medical school, after foundation training, after core training, and specialty training. Doctors are left with the choice of moving home, spending long periods away from their families, or adding a commute onto either end of their shifts. Frequent rotational changes were also highlighted as a source of stress in 'Being a junior doctor'.[1]

A study of anaesthetic trainees elucidated worrying data regarding the reality of fatigue among medical professionals and the effect that it can have, particularly with regards to the demands of commuting. Around 57% of anaesthetic trainees have experienced a crash or near miss when driving home after a night shift, and 84% said that they had felt too tired to drive home.[4] This was not experienced only by motor vehicle drivers; this was also reported by walkers and cyclists.[5] Sadly, these exhausted commutes have resulted in the deaths of several junior doctors in recent years.

The GMC's 2018 national training survey included for the first time a section on fatigue and burnout, and it found that over half of all UK trainees (57%) and half of all UK trainers (50%) who responded to the survey always or often felt worn out at the end of the working day, out of which 32% often or always felt exhausted in the morning at the thought of another day at work.[6]

COMPLAINTS AND LITIGATION

Errare humanum est – but in medicine this sometimes gets turned into accusations of negligence and incompetence. We can be made to see an alter ego in the mirror by these accusations – someone who purposely or incompetently harmed a patient. As a selfless profession dedicated to caring for patients, and also one that is full of perfectionists, accusations such as this can have a significant impact on our mental health. The severity of this issue was highlighted by Clarke et al. in their article 'Suicide should be included among work related causes of death', which examined the messages left behind by junior doctors who had committed suicide over the course of a year. Inevitably, these messages drew a connection between their personal tragedies and the increasing pressures in the NHS.[7]

Complaints against doctors and any legal ramifications that may follow can be extraordinarily stressful. Often, the subject of the complaint is not aware there is an issue until months or years down the line and is forced to recall events that transpired in a different trust or a different part of the country and may have happened in the middle of the night on a busy on-call shift. The process of investigating any incident is long and drawn out, and whereas there is advice available from defence unions that addresses the legal aspects of the case, there is limited pastoral support to tackle the emotional and psychological impact of having one's clinical or interpersonal acumen questioned.

In 2018, Dr Clare Gerarda, former chair of the Royal College of General Practitioners and medical director of the Practitioner Health Programme, published an article, 'Doctors and suicide', in which she detailed the impact of complaints and GMC investigations on doctors' mental health.[8] Bourne et al. also found that doctors who had recently received a complaint of any kind were 77% more likely to suffer from moderate to severe depression than those who had never had a complaint, along with having an increased incidence of suicidal thoughts, sleep difficulties, relationship problems, and physical health problems compared with people who had not received complaints.[9]

In nine years, according to the NHS Practitioner Health Programme, 21 doctors in their care have died, and 52% of these doctors were involved with the GMC. Among current Practitioner Health Programme patients, the GMC is involved in around 10% of cases. Between 2005 and 2013, 28 doctors died through suicide or suspected suicide while undergoing GMC investigation.[8–10]

Unfortunately, complaints and litigation are an increasing feature of life as a doctor, as demonstrated by data from the NHS Litigation Authority (Figure 3.1). Not only is this often an incredible source of stress for individual doctors concerned, but the systemic financial cost is enormous, totalling a staggering £1764.7 million in 2016–2017.[11]

The complaints process is important. It allows patients that haven't received satisfactory care to voice their concerns and should lead to improvements in patient care, but even when complaints are baseless or entirely unfounded, they require a formal response and an investigation. This can be time-consuming and lead to feelings of exasperation, resentment, or embarrassment. Furthermore, recent moves to criminalise medical errors, notably in the case of Dr Bawa-Garba (a trainee paediatrician who was convicted of manslaughter following the death of a child from sepsis), have only heightened the sense of fear that many doctors feel around the possibility of making errors.

NEGATIVE MEDIA PORTRAYAL

Healthcare and the NHS are two topics of almost feverish interest in the UK, and it is rare to see a news bulletin or read a newspaper in which there is not one or more health stories featured prominently. Unfortunately, all too often the focus of these stories is negative and, even if the stories are about systemic failures, it is almost impossible not to feel some personal hurt when the system we work so hard

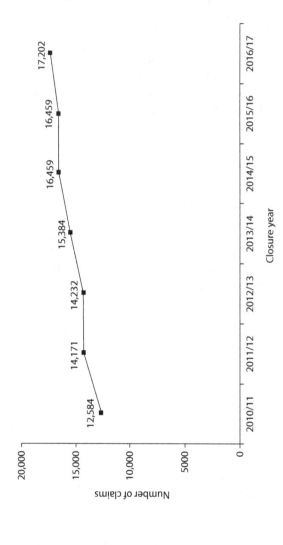

Figure 3.1 The total number of clinical and non-clinical claims closed from 2010–2011 to 2015–2016. (Reproduced from NHS Resolution: Annual Report and Accounts 2016/17. © NHS Resolution.)

to sustain is denigrated. For example, a survey of GPs leaving the medical profession found that over 63% of them cited a negative media portrayal as partly responsible for their decision to leave.[12]

Junior doctors have been directly targeted by mainstream media outlets in recent years, notably in the junior doctors' strikes of 2016 when *The Sun* newspaper ran its 'Moet Medics' campaign which sought to portray junior doctors as louche hedonists by mining their social media feeds for pictures of them on holiday or enjoying themselves with friends. The effect of this negativity can be truly morale-sapping.[13]

With a 24-hour news feed and news appearing on platforms as ubiquitous as the phones in our pockets, the effect of negative media portrayal can feel utterly inescapable.

POLITICAL INTERFERENCE

Over the last three decades, the NHS has undergone a total of 15 major structural reforms.[14] The service is a political football that successive governments remodel and re-mould according to their political whims. The most recent of these major reforms was driven by the 2012 Health and Social Care Act and cost, by conservative estimates, around £1.5 billion to implement. It was so badly thought through and delivered that the King's Fund almost immediately commissioned a report about what had happened, entitled 'Never Again'.[15]

At a system level, these reorganisations can be wasteful, time-consuming, and disruptive, but they also have an impact at an individual level as long-standing departmental and human relationships are broken down by the reshuffles. This can introduce friction into our working world where there was no friction before, and the sense of imposition that these changes bring with them can breed intense resentment, leading to the cynicism and dissatisfaction typical of burnout.

Services may be restructured according to political expediency rather than medical evidence, and thus we see schemes such as tick-box dementia screening for patients during acute hospital admissions, even though there is little evidence of either short- or long-term benefit to the patients as a result of this. Similarly, the four-hour wait in A&E is a politically motivated target that arguably undermines proper triage and the imperative of clinical need and, as a result, creates its own enormous stresses.

There is a tension at the heart of the NHS. As a tax payer–funded institution, the government of the day is rightfully held accountable for its functioning, but this also makes it a convenient tool for vote winning. Plans are frequently made according to the election cycle and what is politically expedient is usually not medically appropriate, and this continual butting of heads, a battle almost inevitably won by those holding the purse strings, can be incredibly draining.

CONCLUSION

Over the last two chapters, we have discussed the stresses that are inherent, and to some extent unavoidable, in the work of being a doctor and also those stresses that are put upon us by the institutions that regulate and monitor us which can often feel excessive, even unnecessary.

Over the following few chapters, we will discuss how we can address these issues both as an individual and at the level of local and national system change. These stressors can be influenced, changed, and adapted to; we just need the will to do this and the knowledge of how to make this happen.

REFERENCES

1. Royal College of Physicians. December 2016. *Being a Junior Doctor – Experiences from the Front Line of the NHS*. Royal College of Physicians.
2. Spooner S et al. 25 October 2017. How do workplaces, working practices and colleagues affect UK doctors' career decisions? A qualitative study of junior doctors' career decision making in the UK. *BMJ Open.* 7: e018462, doi: 10.1136/bmjopen-2017-018462.
3. Rimmer A. 1 December 2016. Workloads threaten to undermine doctors' training, GMC finds. *BMJ.* 355: i6495, doi: 10.1136/bmj.i6495.

4. McClelland L et al. 2017. A national survey of the effects of fatigue on trainees in anaesthesia in the UK. *Anaesthesia*. (Jul), doi: 10.1111/anae.13965, pmid:28681546.

5. Rimmer A. 7th July 2017. *BMJ*. 358: j3328, doi: 10.1136/bmj.j3328.

6. Rimmer A. 9th July 2018. Employers must tackle high level of burnout among trainees, says GMC. *BMJ*. 362: k3018, doi: 10.1136/bmj.k3018.

7. Clarke R et al. 2017 May 26. Suicide should be included among work related causes of death. *BMJ*. 357: j2527, doi: 10.1136/bmj.j2527.

8. Gerada C. April 2018. Doctors and suicide. *Br J Gen Pract*. 68(669): 168–169.

9. Bourne T et al. 2015. The impact of complaints procedures on the welfare, health and clinical practise of 7926 doctors in the UK: A cross-sectional survey. *BMJ Open*. 4: e006687.

10. Horsfall S. 2014. *Doctors Who Commit Suicide While under GMC Fitness to Practice Investigation*. London: General Medical Council.

11. NHS Resolution: Annual Report and Accounts 2016/17.

12. Doran N et al. Feb 2016. Lost to the NHS: A mixed methods study of why GPs leave practice early in England. *Br J Gen Pract*. 66(643): e128–e135.

13. Staten A. 10th September 2014. Stop this Pernicious NHS-Bashing. The Independent.

14. Walshe K. 2010. Reorganisation of the NHS in England. *BMJ*. 341: c3843.

15. King's Fund. 2012. Never Again? The Story of the Health and Social Care Act 2012.

4

Burnout in medical school

JONATHAN C. H. LAU AND
ASHTON BARNETT-VANES

All careers in medicine start with medical school. These institutions are responsible for imparting the skills, knowledge, and training necessary to become competent healthcare professionals. With over 30 recognised schools in the UK, each one distinct from the next, it is clear that medicine has become a widely taught subject, open to both impassioned school-leavers and graduates alike. Yet, getting through medical school is no easy task, as most will attest; it is a serious and arduous undertaking.

When placed against the backdrop of sports, social events, and other extracurricular activities, medical school can feel much the same as any university. However, few studies have such a vocational dimension. Most medical students will graduate and immediately become doctors. Naturally, therefore, there is an expectation of high standards of education, and for medics – who face the prospect of undergoing lifelong learning throughout their career – their time as a student is often the first step to realising the scale of this professional journey.

Given its variety and intensity as a discipline, the culture and practice of medicine is typically associated with high levels of psychological stress, felt not least by medical students. Indeed, there is much evidence that supports the view that a student's mental health is likely to worsen as progress is made towards qualification.[1] Additionally, prevalence rates of depression and anxiety within medical schools may reach as high as 56% – levels exceeding those of similarly aged individuals in the general population.[2] This holds direct implications for dropout rates and more severe consequences such as self-harm or addiction.

In newly qualified doctors, for instance, associations have been found between depressive symptoms and increasing cynicism, as well as lower levels of self-rated health.[3,4] This can ultimately pose a threat to patient safety, as physicians who are under stress have been linked to a diminishing quality of care.[5] Because medical students are the doctors of tomorrow, the need to promote personal wellness during their formative years is critical. Since 2013, guidance released by the General Medical Council (GMC) has helped to raise awareness of such issues, whilst advising medical schools to provide 'appropriate support to students to ensure their health and wellbeing'.[6] Nevertheless, dealing with stress is an inevitable struggle experienced by all students, and for some, the risk of experiencing issues such as burnout and depression remains high despite the availability of supportive services.

However, it is not all doom and gloom! The opportunity to pursue medicine as a career is a unique one with many rewards. This chapter serves as an approachable guide for current and prospective medical students to learn more about, and how to deal with, the stressors they are likely to face at medical school as they train to become future doctors.

THE REALITIES OF MEDICAL SCHOOL

Life at medical school is dynamic and fast-paced. As students, the need to strike a balance between ongoing commitments to work and one's own interests is an constant challenge. Stress is frequently encountered, but it is a natural and unavoidable aspect of the human condition. These experiences, which may be physically, mentally, and emotionally demanding, serve to draw our attention to potentially undesirable or dangerous stimuli. In that sense, they help by prompting us to react and adapt to such situations before they become unmanageable. However, experiencing stress is an uncomfortable sensation in itself and can place a strain on our capacity to cope.

Box 4.1 outlines a number of common sources of stress and divides them into two main groups, those encountered at medical school and those which have a personal dimension. While the list is by no means exhaustive, it is clear that individuals may be affected by multiple stressors at once, and depending on the person, some will be more burdensome than others. This chapter focusses on those regarded as being particularly relevant to medical students.

Preclinical years

Medicine requires students to learn considerable amounts of information in relatively short intervals. Stretched for time, a common question for medical students is 'Will *this* come up in our exams?' Further, new modes of teaching or the demands of transitioning into clinical environments (discussed later) may exacerbate the feeling of not being in sufficient control of your learning and progress. This is not helped by the lack of a universal syllabus for medicine, which may vary between medical schools or year group and thus necessitates devising one's own approach to the subject with little or no reassurance until exam results day.

While sitting through lectures may be preferred by some, others may wish to see patients at the earliest opportunity. With each successive year, there is also increased emphasis on so-called self-directed study skills, particularly as teaching becomes less

BOX 4.1: Common sources of stress at medical school

ACADEMIC STRESSORS (ALL YEARS)

- Increased scholastic workload and difficulty compared with secondary school
- Competition from peers encourages high standard of attainment
- High-stakes examinations (with no possibility of retakes in some cases)
- Unfamiliarity with essay-based assessments
- Frustration with rigidity of multiple-choice assessments/ single best answer
- Need to distinguish oneself by partaking in other forms of study (e.g. research)

CLINICAL STRESSORS (CLINICAL YEARS)

- New environment that brings students closer to actual front-line duties as a doctor
- No control over the types of patients seen
- No control over the quality of supervision
- Administrative errors with timetables, locations, etc.
- Some junior doctors and also some senior doctors may act as poor role models
- Reduced holidays compared with preclinical years

SOCIAL STRESSORS (PERSONAL)

- Loss of contact with friends and family
- Loss of contact with those who have dropped out or are retaking the year
- Loneliness and possible segregation
- Ongoing day-to-day interactions with individuals who do not share same values/beliefs, particularly when on the ward
- Relationship issues involving partners, flatmates (who may also be medics), etc.

PSYCHOLOGICAL STRESSORS (PERSONAL)

- Unrealistic expectations
- Neuroticism

FAMILIAL STRESSORS (PERSONAL)

- Parental pressure
- Family illness

FINANCIAL STRESSORS (PERSONAL)

- Burden of student loans
- Responsibility to others, such as partner or children, in some cases
- Ongoing commitments to part-time employment

SPIRITUAL STRESSORS (PERSONAL)

- Core beliefs may be shaken, questioned, or disregarded with little or no time available to address them personally and allow for spiritual growth

structured, favouring those with independent learning styles. Moreover, having assessments on a regular basis, each with their own distinct formats, such as multiple-choice and written examinations, requires getting used to, especially if they have not been encountered before (or neglected as is usually the case with essays!). Finally, the fierce level of competition amongst peers adds an additional level of stress and ties closely with a number of personal or psychological stressors that are common amongst medical students.

Clinical years

Finishing preclinical medicine can feel like a huge achievement; the learning you've acquired would be sufficient to earn a bachelor's degree in most other scientific endeavours. However, this is just the halfway point. Entering the clinical environment for the first time as a student can be overwhelming.

First, you have to navigate what is essentially a professional working environment replete with office politics, occupational hazards and the steady flow of new, complex, and sometimes uncooperative patients. It takes years to become accustomed to these factors. For medical students, the sense of being hamstrung is a constant source of frustration. Initially, you're able to perform simple clinical tasks, but not yet experienced enough to contribute meaningfully to patient management. As you progress through the years, your ability to contribute more to the clinical team increases; however, so too do your learning commitments.

While being on the ward can serve as excellent preparation for life as a doctor, most students still find themselves investing considerable amounts of energy outside of this 'contact time' to acquire and maintain the clinical knowledge necessary to pass exams. Balancing these two competing demands is stressful, and students can often become occupied by it, for example arriving on consultant ward rounds, but skipping menial ward tasks and instead going to the library. As a result, most medical schools now require students to provide evidence of their participation in clinical environments, either with sign-off sheets or lists of tasks they are expected to perform. Suffice to say, getting on top of these requirements early should be a priority; students can find themselves under considerable stress as exams close in and they're still chasing uncommon procedures on the ward or in theatre.

While on the ward, it is common for medical students to feel isolated and unsupported. Senior doctors, while mindful of your existence, are busy, stressed, and managing their own workloads. Students therefore often find themselves having to work hard to derive learning value out of their day, particularly when no structured teaching is taking place. Many days end without a clear sense of achievement or learning, and this can adversely impact student esteem or confidence.

Finally, the emotional strain of the clinical environment should not be underestimated. Students will see patients who recover well and head home. They will also see tragic cases, cases in which unexpected outcomes occur, cases in which very young or very old people are unable to recover, and so on. Almost all medical students will witness someone die or be present in the immediate aftermath of death. This process, particularly when seen for the first time, can impact significantly on one's emotional state.

BURNOUT IN MEDICAL SCHOOL

Although medics may face myriad issues throughout their studies, it is reassuring to note that the vast majority go on to pass each year and eventually qualify. For some, however, the constant pressure may be too much to handle effectively, resulting in a number of adverse outcomes, be it anxiety, depression, or other symptoms that fall under the umbrella of 'burnout'. Insofar as doctors are concerned, burnout adversely affects the relationship with the patient; for students, this can amount to a similar effect or, at the very least, an unwillingness to commit further to their studies, which can be detrimental to their future fitness to practice.

Stress and the potential for experiencing burnout should be accepted as natural aspects of life that cannot be eliminated. Although facing up to this reality is never easy, ignoring it will not make it any less true. Indeed, it is always better to recognise, confront, and subsequently manage stressful situations in such a way that allows one to avoid the negative consequences associated with it.

Coping

As shown in Box 4.2, there are a number of individual precepts/ actions that one may take to better handle stress and avoid burnout. Here, we will explore some of these further within the context of medical school.

First and foremost is the importance of upholding a positive, can-do attitude. Although university will invariably bring new challenges and setbacks, all students would do well to remember that by being admitted into medical school, they have already demonstrated their enthusiasm and potential to complete the course. The trick, as students, is to discover how best they can realise this potential within the constraints of their programme (Figure 4.1). Unfortunately, there is no easy answer to this, as every student's approach will be influenced by a range of personal factors, such as differing learning styles and varying degrees of interest for

BOX 4.2: Student support actions

- Identify and prioritise activities based on personal core values
- Adopt a healthy lifestyle – with good sleep hygiene, regular exercise, and relevant health check-ups
- Maintain good friendships or relationships with others
- Use peer support systems
- Keep a sense of humour
- Take regular, scheduled vacations
- Recognise that help is always available (e.g. Nightline)

specific topics. Yet, among the most capable students, in addition to optimism, other key traits include having good organisational skills (notably time management), maintaining a social network of close friends and family, a willingness to participate, patience, confidence to test or push their own limits, and, most importantly, not being afraid to back down or ask for help.

Maintaining enthusiasm for a course which may last up to six years is challenging. At one time or another, all medical students

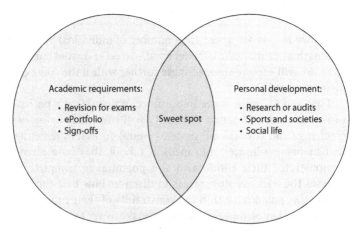

Figure 4.1 Maintaining a healthy balance.

have questioned if this is the course or career that is right for them. However, there are many opportunities available for students during training to broaden their horizons. During the preclinical years, when course structure remains fairly rigid, it may help to draw links to clinical practice to help maintain interest and contextualise why they're learning. For the latter clinical years, where teaching becomes more flexible, opportunities may be taken to advance or hone an interest in a particular field or topic area. This could be through research, audits, or deeper clinical engagement on the ward or clinic or in theatre.

Managing expectations

The highly competitive nature of medical school – and medicine at large – is a source of stress that takes time to internalise. Although competitiveness is a strong motivator for academic achievement, this can lead to excessive levels of overwork with little perceived return. Students should bear in mind that it is more than sufficient to achieve a passing grade without having to idealise oneself as a 'top student'. The reality is that performance in medical school forms but one, albeit essential, part of a professional portfolio, which can be readily boosted by demonstrating keenness in other academic pursuits (e.g. research) or extracurricular activities.

Despite what others may say, the world of medicine offers an incredible breadth of choice, and tailoring professional development in a fair and balanced way carries more weight than prioritising academic excellence. Indeed, all qualifying medics bear the same letters as their contemporaries, and each are expected to perform the same duties to an acceptable standard as the next; it is this same standard that students must remember they are striving towards, nothing beyond or beneath it. As such, many of the essential qualities that make a good doctor cannot be measured by exams alone.

Seeking help

There are times where, despite great effort or adaptation, students become burnt out. This experience, as discussed above, may manifest in differing ways. Its impacts, however, will be typical, whether or not it is noticed by yourself, or a colleague or friend, is irrelevant. If you're not coping, it's essential you act. This can be through your university or outside of it.

At university, your personal tutor, mentor, or dean will be ready to listen and support. They will have likely seen burnout before and can provide a wealth of advice and suggestions on how to help steer yourself back on track. Universities also run excellent counselling and support services which are at your disposal and at which you can raise any issue that's affecting you. Outside of medical school, your general practitioner, counsellor or even a trusted friend will be able to offer advice and support. Remember, if you're experiencing crisis, the Samaritans are available 24 hours a day, as are emergency departments of local hospitals: you never need to suffer in silence.

It is very uncommon for medical students to drop out on account of stress or burnout, but it does happen. While the decision is not to be made lightly, there are a range of options if study is getting on top of you. Each university has their own procedures, and your deans will be best placed to advise you. Regardless, it is important to take time to undergo a period of personal reflection and understand or appreciate the factors that have brought you to this stage. This can mean the difference between completing the course but ultimately not practicing, taking a year or two out, transferring to another course, or leaving medicine altogether. Importantly, the final decision lies with you and you alone, as you are the best judge to determine what is best.

CONCLUSION

Given the range of issues impacting on the life of a medical student, it is not surprising that medicine is regarded as one of the most challenging courses to undertake. From the student's perspective, factors associated with stress often meld together to give the feeling of being overworked. Excessive levels of time pressure, responsibility, and expectations, coupled with inadequate levels of support, can stretch students. Clinical stressors, namely a professional working environment, the sense of being inadequately equipped to be effective in it, the emotional dimension of patient contact, and competing self-directed learning priorities, make the latter years particularly challenging. However, they can be immensely rewarding and constitute a rite of passage for many doctors.

Overall, the process of learning medicine is formidable, but this should hardly be surprising given its scope and the career you're set to follow. And yet, despite all, it should never feel insurmountable. Throughout this chapter, we have evaluated the main sources of stress faced by students and the effects it can have. However, we have also discussed ways of recognising burnout, rekindling enthusiasm, and managing stress. Most importantly, we have attempted to demonstrate how it is possible to view each stressor as having a logical basis and how these may be used to prompt students to behave differently when confronting them. In essence, effectively dealing with stress strengthens students' abilities to cope and manage with future problems and steels them for future success.

ACKNOWLEDGEMENTS

The authors wish to thank C. P. F. Travers, RUMS Vice President (Sports and Societies), for insightful discussions and critical review of the manuscript.

REFERENCES

1. Levine RE, Litwins SD, Frye AW. 2006. An evaluation of depressed mood in two classes of medical students. *Acad Psychiatry.* 30(3): 235–237.
2. Dyrbye LN, Thomas MR, Shanafelt TD. 2006. Systematic review of depression, anxiety, and other indicators of psychological distress among U.S. and Canadian medical students. *Acad Med.* 81(4): 354–373.
3. West CP, Tan AD, Habermann TM, Sloan JA, Shanafelt TD. 2009. Association of resident fatigue and distress with perceived medical errors. *JAMA – J Am Med Assoc.* 302(12): 1294–300.

4. Yi MS et al. 2007. Self-rated health of primary care house officers and its relationship to psychological and spiritual well-being. *BMC Med Educ.* 7: 9.
5. Firth-Cozens J, Greenhalgh J. 1997. Doctors' perceptions of the links between stress and lowered clinical care. *Soc Sci Med.* 44(7): 1017–1022.
6. General Medical Council. 2015. Promoting excellence: Standards for medical education and training.

5

Changing the way we work

ADAM STATEN

Given the demographic changes taking place around the developed world, it seems unlikely that the pressures experienced both by individual doctors and by healthcare systems are going to lessen in the short or medium term. Therefore, whole systems and the doctors that work within them are going to have to adapt to cope with these increasing pressures to avoid catastrophic levels of physician burnout.

Just as these pressures have an impact at individual and system levels, so we should seek to implement changes to the way we work at these different levels. Both organisational change and individual strategies for coping with workload stress have been shown to help doctors and medical students avoid burnout, but it is the changes that can be made at the organisational level that have been shown to be of greatest benefit.[1] Making changes at the organisational level also acknowledges that the problem of burnout is systemic, with individuals suffering because of the system in which they work, and therefore this systemic problem demands a systemic response. However, system change requires time and resource, so students and doctors must also focus on smaller changes that they can make for themselves immediately.

PERSONAL COPING STRATEGIES

Progressing through medical school without developing ways of managing stress is a near impossibility; indeed most people will already have learned to cope with significant stress as part of the process of securing a place at medical school. The coping strategies that most people develop are largely dependent on personality type, personal experience, and preference, but not all coping strategies are equally effective. Many of us have developed coping strategies that may ultimately prove to be inadequate to cope with the increasing demands of study and work as we progress through our careers.

A study examining the personal coping strategies of doctors found that, at work, doctors' coping strategies are encompassed by five major themes. These themes include simply soldiering on through whatever work is thrown at them, talking things through with colleagues, humour, taking a time out, and simply ignoring the stress. Most doctors in the study talked of simply soldiering on or trying to ignore the stress; however, these strategies, perhaps predictably, were ultimately associated with higher levels of emotional exhaustion. These are avoidant strategies, coping strategies that rely on denying the reality of the situation and do not aim to tackle the root cause of the stress. For this reason they can only ever offer temporary relief and will inevitably be inadequate if the stress persists. It is, therefore, not surprising that these coping strategies are associated with higher levels of burnout in the long run.[2]

Those strategies that rely on denial can also be described as forms of 'protective withdrawal'. Protective withdrawal is a valid means of coping with a difficult situation, and many people adopt this strategy: sitting tight and waiting for the situation to change. Problems arise when the situation doesn't change.

Protective withdrawal contrasts to coping mechanisms employed by those people who actively seek to ameliorate the situation, people known in the literature as 'change agents'.[3] Given that those doctors who adopt more proactive coping strategies are least likely to burn out, these are the strategies that we should seek to develop for ourselves.

Making plans of action was identified as one of the more effective coping strategies to manage stress. This might be as simple as writing up a jobs list and identifying which jobs are a priority at the start of the working day, or might involve more significant steps such as identifying your direct lines of management and working out who you can contact to bring about necessary change. In either case, the key element is taking active steps to take control of the situation. Even if actually gaining control is a distant aim, identifying how control might be gained is itself a psychologically worthwhile activity.

Talking things through with colleagues is another effective coping strategy, and one that shouldn't be beyond even the most busy doctor or student. Discussing emotionally challenging situations might be done in a formal situation such as a Balint group or Schwartz Round (of which more later), but could equally be achieved by making the time to sit with a colleague and vent over a cup of coffee. This is a positive step in helping you to identify what the problems are, gaining the benefit of someone else's experiences of the same issues, and so working out how better to manage the stress in the future.

Unfortunately, the stresses of work have a habit of following us home, and so we all need ways to relieve our stress away from the workplace. The same study that investigated physician coping strategies at work found that the most popular coping strategies used by doctors to relieve themselves of stress at home include exercise, talking to a partner, spending time with the family, or having some quiet time alone. These were all found to be helpful and were more common than less-effective coping strategies such as using alcohol to unwind or simply carrying on working at home.[2] This again demonstrates that active strategies are more effective than passive strategies, and this study also underlines the intuitive fact that, to be happy and effective at work, we need a good work-life balance that also allows us to be happy at home.

When workload is high and people are feeling stressed there is a temptation to hunker down and just try to survive. This is not sustainable because the stresses in healthcare are not going away. For a sustainable career it is essential to actively carve out protected time to spend with friends and family, undertake hobbies, and take exercise.

TEAM BUILDING

With the move away from traditional firm structures in hospital and towards shift-based work, junior doctors working within modern healthcare systems can experience the paradox of feeling very isolated despite being apparently surrounded by colleagues.

People form bonded groups after sharing experiences that are personally shaping, or emotionally impactful, in some way.[4] The more of these experiences we share, both positive and negative, the more bonded we become, and the more bonded we become, the better we cooperate and work together.[5] Whilst the old firm structure was by no means perfect, it is self-evident that the daily sharing of the highs and lows of the on-call was an effective means of getting people to share emotionally challenging experiences and so bonding them together as a team. A disjointed shift rota, by contrast, may mean that we never work again with someone with whom we have been through a difficult shift. Therefore we do not develop as a team.

In the absence of natural team development in this way, it is arguably more important than ever that junior doctors work at building teams from which they can draw mutual support. This was highlighted in the Royal College of Physicians report 'Being a Junior Doctor: Experiences from the Front Line of the NHS', in which doctors reported the breakdown of the team as a key factor in low morale.[6] Building a team does not require muddy afternoons on an assault course or hours of group hugs and navel gazing, but the simple principles of team building can be built into every shift.

Teams are most effective when they have clear roles and responsibilities and know what their shared goals are.[7] This can be achieved at a fairly basic level simply by meeting as a team at the beginning of a shift, identifying who is who in the team and agreeing how you are going to work together.

Day to day, short coffee breaks to make chitchat and discuss difficult problems should not be seen as a luxury, but as a necessity to provide more effective patient care and make stress more bearable for doctors. However difficult it may seem to find five minutes to get together, it is vital to maintaining a healthy and effective team. This can and should be re-enforced digitally by using platforms such as WhatsApp™ or Facebook™ (although clearly patient identifiable information shouldn't be shared on insecure services).

It is for this same reason that the institution of the doctors' mess, both as a physical space for coming together and as a concept to encourage socialising, should be defended. In this respect, it is heartening to see the Royal College of Physicians (RCP) promote a scheme of 'chief registrars' in whose remit is encouraging the engagement and morale of junior doctors within the hospital, as well as developing our future medical leaders.[8]

ORGANISATIONAL CHANGES

There are numerous interventions that can be made at an organisational level that can reduce the chance of junior-doctor burnout, including anti-bullying policies, the introduction of flexible working hours (where possible), promoting mentoring programmes, and the use of leadership programmes, such as the RCP chief registrar programme.[9] Due to the complexity of introducing programmes such as these into even moderately sized organisations, the evidence base is limited, but the evidence that exists suggests that these interventions are effective.

Team building, as discussed above, is intended to improve the social support of doctors at work, but this is too important to be the responsibility of individual doctors, and so organisations should build mechanisms to weave this social support into the fabric of working life. Providing increased levels of social support, whether that is with mentoring schemes, peer support, or simply allowing people the time to chat and engage with one another, has been shown to decrease symptoms of post-traumatic stress disorder (PTSD) and depression, as well as having a positive impact on physical functioning and health. Interestingly, there also seems to be a positive association between giving social support, for example by being the mentor, and mental and physical health, and so programmes of peer, or near-peer mentorship should also be explored.[10]

Within medicine, we have traditionally not prepared ourselves well for the emotional demands of our jobs. Organisations such as the military and police now invest in preparatory training with the aim of readying their employees for the experience of stressful situations and the impact these experiences are likely to have on them psychologically.[10] For example, British soldiers fighting in Afghanistan during the early part of this century went through Trauma Risk Management (TRiM) training to ready them for the psychological aftermath of combat. The lessons learnt in this preparatory training were then refreshed immediately after particularly difficult incidents. This helped to normalise and validate the natural reactions to traumatic experiences, such as difficulty sleeping and intrusive thoughts, in a way that the doctrine of 'detached concern' within medicine does not.

Preparatory training is heavily based around the creation of realistic scenarios. In medicine, we already do this by role play, trauma moulages, and basic life support (BLS) training, but the focus is almost always on the immediate clinical scenario rather than the psychological aftermath of being involved in these stressful situations.

However, some medical schools in America have set up well-being programmes for medical students with the intention of preparing them for the stress ahead. At Boston Medical School, for example, a programme centred around yoga and meditation was shown to help in promoting resilience, and curriculum changes made at the St Louis University School of Medicine, with the specific aim of preventing burnout, were shown to reduce anxiety and depression amongst students. Similar programmes, with similar successes, were rolled out for new faculty members at the Medical School at Calgary University and for academic physicians at the Mayo Clinic, where the programme was shown to reduce burnout and increase a sense of empowerment in staff.[11]

Just as TRiM training in the army validated post-traumatic psychological experiences, so these medical school programmes normalised the expectation of stress. This helps to shift the problem of burnout from one of being an individual fault to a recognised systemic hazard.

More than just preparing students and junior doctors for stressful situations, organisations should also implement routine sessions whereby staff can discuss the fallout from particularly difficult and demanding patient encounters. Balint groups are one means by which this can be achieved. Named after the Hungarian psychoanalyst who devised them whilst researching his 1957 book *The Doctor, His Patient and the Illness,*[12] Balint groups provide a non-judgemental forum for doctors to discuss cases which have provoked anxiety in them and that they have found difficult to deal with. Balint groups are common, indeed almost universal, during GP and psychiatry training but are little used in other specialties.

Similarly, the Schwartz Round is a structured forum where staff from all disciplines can come together and focus on the emotional impact (rather than the clinical difficulty) of patient interactions. Ideally carried out on a monthly basis and lasting about an hour, a panel of around four staff members, usually a mix of clinical and non-clinical, begin the discussion which may be around a particular case or a theme such as 'a patient I will never forget' before opening it up for reflective discussion for the wider group. The benefit of Schwartz Rounds is in making staff feel more supported, recognising the contributions that different staff members make to patient care, and sharing the experience of being emotionally impacted by caring for patients.[13]

MANAGING CONFLICT

Working within a stressful, resource-limited environment inevitably leads to conflict in the workplace. Conflict is counterproductive and adds to the stress of an already stressful situation. Evidence suggests that conflict is seen by many doctors in training as a key influence in lack of job satisfaction and low morale.[14] Whilst medical schools place an increasing emphasis on communication skills, this is largely focused at managing difficult doctor–patient interactions and far less so on the conflicts that can emerge amongst staff, this despite a plethora of lay literature about managing conflict in the workplace. In general, it is simply expected that junior doctors will learn to be skilled conflict managers as their career progresses.

Whereas disagreement can fuel debate and may lead to useful progress, conflict is a damaging and negative entity and the progression from disagreement to conflict may result from pre-existing underlying tensions in the workplace. The development of conflict can be seen as occurring in four phases: first is frustration, second is the rapid conceptualisation or rationalisation of the cause for your frustration (which may not be accurate), phase three is acting out behaviours to address the perceived cause of the frustration, and the final phase is a destructive or damaging outcome as a result of these behaviours.[15] For example, you may be frustrated that your colleague won't answer his bleep, you rationalise this situation by assuming he is being lazy, you act upon your frustration by accusing him of being lazy, and the outcome is him disengaging from you and your job being harder as a result.

We have all experienced situations where a frustration has rapidly led to a regrettable action that has only served to heighten tension and conflict. Common sources of frustration for doctors include communication difficulties (e.g. unanswered beeps or phone calls), information overload (e.g. a caseload of too many patients or very complex patient problems), ambiguous instructions or ambiguous job roles (i.e. 'whose responsibility is this?'), inadequate information (e.g. patient notes or results not available), or wrong information (e.g. poor handover).[16] Recognising why we are coming into conflict and considering the underlying factors that may be aggravating the situation is useful in working out how to handle it. It is therefore important to resist the urge to leap to a conclusion about why we feel frustrated, and think through the issue logically. In the example above, rather than jumping to the conclusion that your colleague is being lazy, you resist the urge to accuse him of being workshy and instead find him and find out that he is just as busy as you and has been unable to answer his bleep because of this. This discussion leads you to find that you have workload problems in common, and together you create a plan to help both of you deal with the excess workload more effectively.

Saltman, O'Dea, and Kidd describe how conflict can be handled in four ways: avoidance (denying the conflict exists), accommodation (letting the other party have their way), competition, or collaboration. An awareness of these four strategies is useful in order to recognise how we handle our conflicts and why this may or may not result in the outcomes we want. The first two strategies are often expedient ways to diffuse a situation but are likely to potentiate frustration in the long run, or simply leave conflict unresolved. Competition may be a useful way of succeeding in an environment with limited resources but runs counter to efforts to build teams and may ultimately foster resentment and fuel further conflict. Collaboration is perhaps the best means of resolving conflict to allow sustainable change and productivity, but it is time consuming, draining, and difficult to make work if there are already pre-existing problems with the relationship between interested parties.[15]

Each of these four ways of managing conflict has its place, but when we encounter conflict, we should be conscious of which strategy we are choosing to use and aware of the benefits and risks of our chosen strategies. Handled well, conflicts can be diffused and lead to increased productivity, group cohesion, and resolution of problems. Handled badly, conflict leads to division, ill will, and decreased productivity.

CONCLUSION

Work as a junior doctor is difficult and stressful and will always be so, but these stresses can be managed by learning to work differently as individuals, work better as teams, seek ways of integrating stress management into the work environment, and learning how better to handle conflicts in the workplace.

REFERENCES

1. West CP, Dyrbye LN, Erwin PJ, Shanafelt TD. 2016. Interventions to prevent and reduce physician burnout: A systematic review and meta-analysis. *Lancet*. England. 388(10057): 2272–2281.
2. Lemaire JB, Wallace JE. 2010. Not all coping strategies are created equal: A mixed methods study exploring physicians' self reported coping strategies. *BMC Health Serv Res*. England. 10: 208.
3. Lown M, Lewith G, Simon C, Peters D. 2015. Resilience: What is it, why do we need it, and can it help us? *Br J Gen Pract*. England. 65(639): e708–10.
4. Newson M et al. 2016. Explaining lifelong loyalty: The role of identity fusion and self-shaping group events. *PLOS ONE*. 11(8): e0160427.
5. Balliet D, Wu J, De Dreu CKW. Ingroup favoritism in cooperation: A meta-analysis. *Psychol Bull*. 140: 1556–1581.
6. Royal College of Physicians. December 2016. *Being a Junior Doctor: Experiences from the Front Line of the NHS*. London: RCP.
7. Royal College of Physicians. 2017. *Improving Teams in Healthcare, Resource 1: Building Effective Teams*. London: RCP.
8. Royal College of Physicians. RCP Chief Registrar Scheme. Available: www.rcplondon.ac.uk/projects/rcp-chief-registrar-scheme. Accessed: 19th August 2018.
9. Murray M, Murray L, Donnelly M. 2016. Systematic review of interventions to improve the psychological well-being of general practitioners. *BMC Fam Pract*. England. 17: 36.
10. Southwick SM, Pietrzak RH, White G. 2011. Interventions to enhance resilience and resilience-related constructs in adults. In Southwick SM, Litz BT, Charney D, Friedman MJ (eds) *Resilience and Mental Health: Challenges Across the Lifespan*. Cambridge: Cambridge University Press. pp. 289–306.

11. Brown GE, Bharwani A, Patel KD, Lemaire JB. 2016. An orientation to wellness for new faculty of medicine members: Meeting a need in faculty development. *Int J Med Educ*. England. 7: 255–60.
12. Balint M. 1957. *The Doctor, His Patient and the Illness*. London: Churchill Livingstone.
13. Point of Care Foundation. Schwartz Rounds. Available: www.pointofcarefoundation.org.uk/our-work/schwartz-rounds/. Accessed: 19th August 2018.
14. Randall CS et al. 1997 Nov-Dec. Factors associated with primary care residents' satisfaction with their training. *Fam Med*. 29(10): 730–5.
15. Saltman D, O'Dea N, Kidd M. 2006 Jan. Conflict management: A primer for doctors in training. *Postgrad Med J*. 82(963): 9–12.
16. Gibson C, Cohen B. 2003. *Virtual Teams that Work Creating Conditions for Virtual Team Effectiveness*. 1st ed. San Francisco: Jossey Bass.

6

Finding a voice

ADAM STATEN, DUNCAN SHREWSBURY,
ELIZABETH WATERS-DAPRE AND
BEN BALOGUN

Being unable to control the way we work – lacking decision latitude – is a key factor in burnout. Whilst a high workload may not necessarily cause undue stress, being unable to influence the way you manage that workload is extremely stressful. Working and training within a system as vast as the NHS can make you feel insignificant, and it can feel like changing the system in a way to make your workload more manageable is an ambition completely out of your reach. But there are in fact numerous ways in which to exert some influence, and this chapter explores a few of them.

INFLUENCING THE SYSTEM

DUNCAN SHREWSBURY

The bumper sticker quote 'be the change you want to see' is often attributed, somewhat contentiously, to Ghandi. Whilst the provenance of this phrase is dubious, the sentiment has value and holds some truth.

There is no escaping the fact that working in healthcare is enormously challenging. The environment and demands of the job may well, at times, compromise your wellbeing and sense of self.[1] It is tempting to think, indeed I am convinced, that there is an innate human tendency towards falling into a rut of complaining about, and feeling negative and helpless towards, circumstances that detract from job satisfaction and wellbeing. Reflecting on, and sharing, negative experiences with a supportive group of peers can be therapeutic and beneficial in the right doses. However, there is also immense potential in the opportunities afforded by engaging with organisations to help effect the change that you feel needs to be seen more widely. Engaging with these and helping to create the change you want to see can be both rewarding and restorative. Indeed, taking action in this manner corresponds to the principles of self-determination theory, which suggests that we need autonomy, connection with others, and constructive feedback in order to thrive.[2]

As a student or trainee in medicine, you will find yourself in privileged, as well as challenging, positions. Yes, there are organisations that may feel more task-oriented and driven by targets, evaluation, and seemingly punitive regulation. However, they are outnumbered by the number of people, groups, societies, and organisations that wish to improve conditions in healthcare for the benefit of our patients and our professional colleagues.

In the UK, we are fortunate to have an array of bodies that are concerned with training, development, and standards within the medical profession. This is primarily aimed at ensuring that the organisation and quality of healthcare provision in the country is optimised as much as possible for the benefit of patients and the public.

Royal Colleges, and their faculties, represent the majority of different specialties within medicine. Primary medical training at medical school is the concern of the Medical Schools Council and the General Medical Council. Postgraduate training is overseen by Health Education England, NHS Education for Scotland, the Wales Deanery, and the Northern Ireland Medical and Dental Training Agency. Other related bodies include the British Medical Association, which is primarily concerned with advocacy and representation on behalf of the interests of the profession. Almost all of these organisations will have committees, groups, or bodies within them that provide a structure to represent medical students, trainees, and doctors at various other stages of their careers. These groups will regularly hold elections to recruit new candidates to join and are also often open to people attending to 'observe' meetings, to offer specific input on co-opted matters.

It can often seem difficult to get involved with larger organisations, such as Royal Colleges, but there are often a variety of ways to engage at different career stages, either through formal routes such as representation on committees or by seeking involvement on specific matters either through invitation or by asking to get involved or proposing an idea. In my experience, when someone approaches with an idea, and something that may present a solution to an identified gap, there is usually a healthy amount of interest and enthusiasm from organisations to explore it and bring people on board to help take things forward. That is not to say it is easy, and there is no denying that knowing who to make contact with, as well as good timing, plays an important role in determining how input may be received.

Factors that can help garner support for a new idea include

- Follow Covey's[3] advice and seek to understand first, before being understood. What is the nature of the problem, and what do we already know about it?
- Create a shared understanding of this problem and what the desired alternative would be.
- Involve people in generating ideas for solutions; learn from other disciplines and sectors.

- Put together a formal 'pitch' and present a succinct case for what the central issue is, why it is important, what you are proposing, and why that needs support.
- Work out who you need to know and who you need to have help from. Often this means someone who works 'behind the scenes' that has an understanding of how proposals need to be formatted, which governance structures they need to be approved by, and how to get them there.
- Make information about the background of the work and what it intends to achieve publicly available and easily accessible.
- Keep checking what you are doing with a colleague within the organisation. It is easy to stray outside of lines you are not aware of.

Lastly, enjoy the experience. Such opportunities can enrich your training and provide you with a wealth of additional leadership and project-development experience that will ultimately help you and your patients in the long run. But, perhaps most importantly, take care of yourself. It can be uniquely challenging to lead on something. It can sensitise you to criticism and add pressure when you are already busy. Take time to reflect on your own wellbeing, and learn to allow others to help when needed, or to say no.

THE BMA

The BMA is the doctors' trade union in the UK and, whilst not all doctors are members, it is effectively the voice of the profession. Amongst other things, the BMA acts to influence change at both a local and national level to ensure the highest standards of patient care through appropriate design and delivery of healthcare services, and it aims to protect and push for fair working conditions for doctors. For example, the BMA runs campaigns to push forward the agenda of its members, such as 'Caring, Supportive, Collaborative: a Future Vision for the NHS', which has workforce planning and the inculcation of a supportive culture at its centre. On a smaller scale, local negotiating committees will work with acute trusts to make sure working conditions at individual hospitals are acceptable.

It is with the BMA that the government negotiates on big issues such as contracts and pay; so, for anybody wishing to have influence over some of the biggest issues affecting our profession, the BMA is a key body with which to engage. This is possible at several levels, whether that is local, regional, or national, and BMA committees provide an opportunity to bring about real and tangible changes to improve the working life of doctors.

ACTING AS A BMA REPRESENTATIVE ON THE LOCAL NEGOTIATING COMMITTEE

Elizabeth Dapre

It was probably around the beginning of my FY2 year that I began feeling a little disillusioned. The excitement of being a shiny new doctor was wearing off, and with escalating tension surrounding a new contract for junior doctors which was being imposed by the health secretary, the cracks in the system were beginning to show.

There is no denying that working as a doctor is a hugely daunting and demanding task to begin with, but adding in political tensions, rota gaps, pay freezes, and an ever-increasing strain on the NHS, coupled with a significant financial squeeze, can sometimes make the job feel like an impossible undertaking. There were times I felt like throwing in the towel and returning to my previous job in sales and marketing (these were generally following twelve day stretches of 10–12 hour shifts or when I'd missed yet another birthday, wedding, or family event), but I knew that if I gave up hope of change so early on in my career I would burn out.

I decided that, somehow, I would try to influence change for the better. I wanted to be part of moulding a better professional life for myself and my colleagues, and I finally realised that no amount of complaining to my friends and family over yet another glass of Malbec was going to make any difference. I needed to start influencing change from the *inside*.

There were different ways to tackle this, but the most obvious one was to become an elected British Medical Association representative who sat on the Local Negotiating Committee (LNC) at my trust. By becoming an elected representative within my trust I was able to sit on the LNC alongside senior colleagues, management, and hospital directors (and more recently, of course, the guardian of safe working hours), and so negotiate any local issues which had been raised by my colleagues. Topics have ranged from pay discrepancies and delayed payments, working hours, ability (or inability) to take breaks, rota gaps and escalation processes, patient safety, parking availability, safety of staff getting home out of hours, local accommodation for doctors working extended shifts, general morale amongst doctors, and, more recently, ensuring that junior doctors are engaging with exception reporting and deciding where the resultant fines are most appropriately allocated.

Many doctors often feel that management are 'out of touch' with the challenges that we face on a day-to-day basis, and by taking on this role it gave me the opportunity to raise concerns with managers and the medical director of the hospital directly. In this way, I was able to influence change for the better; positive outcomes included the recruitment of additional staff in certain specialties to alleviate workload, improved communication between junior doctors and management, and a review of payroll systems.

It goes without saying that the more elected representatives that sit on the LNC, the broader the junior doctor reach throughout the trust, and the more concerns can be tackled. Although I wasn't able to fix *everything*, I rather felt a sense of comfort knowing that I was at least doing *something* to push for positive change for myself and my colleagues.

THE ROYAL COLLEGES

There are 24 Royal Colleges and faculties in the UK and Ireland. Their primary role is to ensure the quality and safety of the care provided to our patients by setting the standards for training, designing curricula, and making sure that trainees are monitored and mentored through their careers.

Beyond this, the Royal Colleges are able to provide a coherent and unified voice to represent their specialty, and they can bring the weight of their professional and academic credibility to bear when lobbying governments to bring about change in the system. All Royal Colleges and faculties have trainee committees through which trainees can find a voice to argue for the changes they feel are needed within their own specialty. Engaging with these committees is an opportunity to take control of the issues within a specialty and change training and working conditions for the better.

LESSONS LEARNED FROM A TRAINEE-LED INITIATIVE

Duncan Shrewsbury

It is unfortunately the case that those training and working within the medical profession are at significantly greater risk of mental illness and suicide.[1] At a time when junior doctor morale in the UK was believed to be at a nadir, several cases in which junior doctors had turned to suicide were prevalent in the UK mainstream media. GP trainees on the Royal College of General Practitioners (RCGP) Associates in Training committee wanted to take action to address this issue.

At a February meeting of the whole committee, we developed an idea to support a vision of happy, healthy colleagues, who were able to invest in and maintain their wellbeing. We acknowledged the challenge of stigma around such issues and were wary of adding to the negativity. The idea of trying to achieve change positively prompted us to look wider. Drawing on ideas from positive psychology (literally, the study of how positive outcomes are achieved, rather than the study of psychopathology),[4] we took inspiration from work done in the teaching profession with a campaign called #Teacher5aDay.

Their campaign centred on the five themes that emerged from a systematic review published in 2008,[5] which looked at wellbeing across society. The five themes were connect, be active, take notice, keep learning, and give. We re-deployed this as #GP5aDay (with the blessing from the #Teacher5aDay team).

The teachers had given out 'wellbeing bags' to their colleagues. These bags contained little messages about the campaign and treats that were aligned to the messages, such as tea bags (to *connect* with someone over a cup of tea). Instead of leaflets further highlighting the negativity around working in healthcare at present, we felt the wellbeing bags offered an alternative form of campaign collateral that would help signpost key messages and resources, as well as catalyse conversations when taken by trainees and shared with their peers and colleagues.

Our proposal gained support within the College. The campaign collateral was refined, piloted, and lastly showcased at a council meeting. The feedback was largely positive. The bags had morphed into boxes. The tea bags were still present, but were now joined by a mindfulness colouring book and a gratitude journal (both of which have a growing body of evidence suggesting their utility in mental wellbeing[6–8]).

Separated from the aims and messages of the campaign, an image of the mindfulness colouring book appeared on social media and in the trade press.

Subsequently, general practitioners across the country became enraged at the idea that they may be posted a colouring book to solve the issues that the over-stretched and under-resourced workforce faced. Our objective, and morals, were questioned. The idea of the campaign was challenged. Plans to embark on a wider trial were slowed.

This experience conferred several important lessons: firstly, the adage of not being able to please everyone is so true. Intentions can be misconstrued. When you are in a position of responsibility, seek a wide and diverse range of views and critique to hone your work. Create a shared understanding of the aim that drives your work, ideally during the development stages, and then share this wider. Secondly, in whatever you do, ensure you involve all the right people and observe the right processes along the way. A trail of evidence demonstrating appropriate governance has been observed can become valuable should motives and actions be questioned. Lastly, take time to reflect on your own wellbeing. It behoves you, your patients, and the colleagues you work with and for to be the best version of you that you can be.

FREE OPEN-ACCESS MEDICAL (FOAM) EDUCATION

BEN BALOGUN

Free Open-Access Medical education, or Meducation, is as much an ethos as an educational tool. The idea of FOAM is to have a community of junior doctors sharing resources and information that can constantly be updated and constantly evolve. It is a way for doctors and medical students to share the latest in good practice and to help one another, but it can also be a means of influencing the way we work and train within our specialties.

FOAM provides a forum that allows trainees to share and publish work and openly discuss training issues using social media forums such as Facebook and Twitter. For example, most doctors in training do a lot of individual work, either to fulfil training commitments or in preparation for exams, and the vast majority of this work is not shared, published, or made available for other trainees coming up the ranks. Inevitably, there is duplication of work, and newer trainees often make the same mistakes as their predecessors. Time is a precious commodity to a trainee, so having to produce work or study materials from scratch that may already have been developed by someone else seems a poor use of valuable time. FOAM is a way of stopping this waste.

FOAM is a relatively new concept, and one of the advantages of working with new technology and new media, particularly within the old medical establishments, is that there is a high level of interest from the top. This can give you access to influential people within a specialty and allow you to influence both clinical practice and the delivery of training.

Sharing knowledge, learning about new practice, and airing our opinions with colleagues from around the world improves the way we train and the way we treat our patients, and this enhances job satisfaction and can combat burnout.

LONDONEM.COM: A FOAM INITIATIVE

Ten years post-qualification as a doctor I was nearing the end of my EM training and I needed a break from the gruelling regime of the programme – the shift work, covering the vast curriculum, numerous mandatory courses (one expiring just as you've completed another), the seemingly never-ending exams that you wish you had more time to prepare for. I opted to undertake an Out of Training Programme in which I split my time 50:50 between training and non-training commitments. I decided I wanted to spend the non-training part of my programme looking at using technology to enhance education in emergency medicine, particularly with respect to the use of social media and the vast web resources already out there.

The idea of FOAM, though not new to me, was one that the Royal College of Emergency Medicine hadn't fully appreciated. Yes of course there were educational resources designed by the college which were available online to trainees to help them meet their curriculum needs; however, what was missing was the collaborative and evolutionary element added by FOAM.

Teams of emergency medicine doctors from all over the world were producing great work using various platforms and making these freely available online for consumption at will. This was very attractive to me and the college came on board with the idea and gave me an opportunity to come up with an open online platform for EM trainees. This was the birth of the LondonEM project. Collaborating with a few enthusiastic trainees and allied health colleagues, we are able to set up our own FOAM site – LondonEM.com.

There was interest in the project at a high level within the Royal College of Emergency Medicine (RCEM), for example, for my FOAM fellowship post, I was directly supervised by the then Head of School as well as a Professor of Emergency Medicine. This was not because they were experts on the subject, but rather because they were very interested in its potential and keenly aware of how it could potentially revolutionise medical education and training. For me this also meant easy access to the head of school and therefore some influence – a seat at the proverbial table.

I had a voice, and a strong one, with a lot of interested parties. As a result, I was able to help re-shape delivery of aspects of the curriculum using new media, as well as allowing trainees to submit work done or consumed within this forum as evidence of training and continuing education. This also lead to an honorary lectureship at a prestigious London University to deliver FOAM to post-graduate medics.

On a national level, I was also invited as a faculty member to the Developing Excellence in Medical Education Conference (DEMEC), where I presented to decision makers about the benefits of using FOAM and social media to enhance medical education. I was also sponsored to go on courses and conferences to help enhance this project. So, for me, this time out of training has not only helped recharge my batteries as an EM doctor, it has opened doors that I was never aware were available to me and given me access to decision makers, allowing me to directly influence training and delivery of care.

HARNESSING SOCIAL MEDIA

ADAM STATEN

Nigel Lawson, the former Tory chancellor, once described the NHS as the closest thing that the English have to a religion. The British interest in healthcare is almost obsessive, and it is rare for a news programme or newspaper not to feature health stories prominently. And yet, whilst the NHS remains a revered institution, the coverage of the service, and those who work within it, is relentlessly negative, with journalists spewing vitriol about waiting lists, unavailable treatments, or doctors and nurses who have made mistakes. One study found that this negative media portrayal ranked highly amongst reasons for GPs leaving the profession.[9]

The motivation for such critical coverage is not always obvious but includes the political agenda of particular publications, perceived government pressure on state-funded outlets such as the BBC, and the modern pressures of journalism, in which ratings are king, because publicity is easier to attract with bad news than with good news. Often, the motivation appears to be simple spite.

This endless criticism from the mainstream media can be incredibly demoralising and gives the perception that the general public are at odds with the medical profession, thus undermining the traditional values of the patient–doctor relationship which is reliant on trust and respect in both directions.

Penetrating mainstream media platforms to express a more balanced view or counter the most mindless of the criticism is beyond the reach of most working doctors and medical students, but we are fortunate to have alternative means of expressing our views and reaching a wide audience in the form of social media.

The junior doctors' strike of a few years ago provides a good example of this in action. *The Sun* newspaper ran a campaign during the strikes to undermine the junior doctors, the notorious 'Moet Medics' campaign which sought to portray junior doctors as cosseted sybarites. This cynical campaign was effectively undone by the social media response of junior doctors. Whilst many newspapers and TV programmes sought to portray the strikes in a negative light, the noise on social media made it evident that, in reality, there was overwhelming public support for the protest, and this reinforced the resolve of the juniors and helped to legitimise the strikes.

The beauty of social media, whether that is writing blogs, sending tweets, or posting on social media sites, is that it opens up a two-way dialogue allowing doctors to converse with the public and put across nuanced and detailed arguments. As a result of sharing on social media, a well-written or interesting article can reach an enormous, global audience within minutes of publication, even if the platform on which it initially appears is relatively obscure.

Expressing your thoughts and concerns to other people can be incredibly cathartic but is also a genuinely effective way of getting important messages out to the general public when the mainstream media is too ignorant or too obdurate to do so. There is also potential for this to create a virtuous circle of media coverage as the mainstream media derives much of its content from what is trending on social media, and so these social media messages can percolate into the mainstream narrative.

Social media presents doctors with a great opportunity to educate patients and influence public opinion, and it is public opinion that will ultimately dictate the direction in which services are taken.

REFERENCES

1. Brooks SK, Gerada C, Chalder T. 2011. Review of literature on the mental health of doctors: Are specialist services needed? *J Ment Health.* 20(2): 146–156.
2. Deci EL, Ryan RM. 2011. Chapter 20: Self-determination theory. In Van Lange PAM, Kriglanski AW, Higgins ET (eds) *Handbook of Theories in Social Psychology*, volume 1. Thousand Oaks, CA: SAGE Publications.
3. Covey S. 1989. *The 7 Habits of Highly Effective People.* New York: Free Press.
4. Styles C. 2011. *Brilliant Positive Psychology: What Makes Us Happy, Optimistic, and Motivated.* Harlow: Pearson Education.
5. Aked J, Marks N, Cordon C, Thompson S. 2008. Five ways to wellbeing: a report presented to the Foresight Project on communicating the evidence base for improving people's well-being. *New Economics Foundation.* Available: http://b.3cdn.net/ nefoundation/8984c5089d5c2285ee_t4m6bhqq5.pdf. Accessed: 19th August 2018.
6. Emmons RA, Crumpler CA. 2000. Gratitude as a human strength: Appraising the evidence. *J Soc Clin Psychol.* 19(1): 56–59.
7. Van der Vennet R, Serice S. 2012. Can colouring mandalas reduce anxiety? A replication study. *Art Therapy.* 29(2): 87–92.
8. Shapiro SL, Brown KW, Biegel GM. 2007. Teaching self-care to caregivers: Effects of mindfulness-based stress reduction on the mental health of therapists in training. *Train Educ Prof Psychol.* 1(2): 105–115.
9. Doran N, et al. Feb 2016. Lost to the NHS: A mixed methods study of why GPs leave practice early in England. *Br J Gen Pract.* 66(643): e128–e135.

7

Finding the right career

ADAM STATEN

A medical career can feel like a treadmill. *Modernising Medical Careers* was introduced in 2005 in the UK in order to standardise training for doctors to produce a predictable flow of newly qualified doctors in at one end and a predictable flow of consultants and GPs out at the other. This created a feel that a medical career should be an inexorable progression, a ladder that you climb alongside your peers and from which you shouldn't fall off.

There is plenty of evidence to show that doctors at every level have sought ways to jump off the treadmill and diversify their careers with FY3 years, periods of research or further study, or time abroad, but it remains the case that most doctors focus largely on the purely clinical aspect of their role with an ultimate progression into a specialty consultant post in a more or less traditional role.

The world of medicine is, however, a very diverse place, and medical professionals are very adaptable people. There are numerous roles that doctors can fulfil both inside and outside of the NHS, either as an alternative to a traditional, clinical career, or as complementary to that career. This variety of work can be a powerful tonic to the stresses of the day job, giving us the opportunity to think differently, work in different ways, and find different ways to gain personal satisfaction from our careers.

7.1

Researcher

DAVID N. NAUMANN

During a doctor's career, there are opportunities to pause clinical training in order to take some time out to undertake research as part of a higher degree – for example an MD or PhD. This is usually designated as 'Out of Programme for Research' (OOPR). During this period, the doctor will become a student at a university and will be expected to plan, design, and implement a research project that will form the basis of a doctorate thesis. Their thesis will be expected to contain novel data that 'adds' to the scientific understanding of that subject. An OOPR is an opportunity for both professional and personal development and offers a change in working pattern to that otherwise experienced by junior doctors during training.

WHY GET INVOLVED IN RESEARCH?

Taking some time out of training for research is one way of experiencing a new style and tempo of work, with more autonomy and flexibility than might be expected during clinical training. It may also be an opportunity to explore your academic interests and, of course, expand your CV. People choose to do research for a number of reasons; some might have a particular interest in a certain topic, some may want to explore a different career pathway, some might simply want a change or a break from training.

As a junior doctor in training, you may find yourself mentally saturated whilst working relatively long hours that include weekends and nights, leaving very little room for reading about the latest evidence or thoughtful exploration of scientific ideas. Taking some time out of training to undertake research is a perfect opportunity to allow for more time and capacity to think, take stock of your situation, and slow things down in life. That's not to say that research means doing less work, but it usually means more sociable working hours, more time to read and learn new ideas, and a unique opportunity to design and undertake your own research.

One of the most appealing aspects of a new working style is that it can be a refreshing change, and one that offers variety to an otherwise unidirectional career path. After all, as many Consultants and GPs will tell you, there's really no rush to finish training, and sometimes it is worth adding something extra to your training that you might not necessarily be able to do later. If research is something that you are seriously considering, then you are already halfway there!

I think it's also important to mention here one reason *not* to go into research. Some doctors may be tempted to embark on a higher degree because of a belief that it will be necessary to get a consultant job or to get into specialty training. If this becomes the only reason that a doctor undertakes a higher degree, it is likely that it will not be as enjoyable or rewarding and may even be counterproductive. I've spoken to some doctors who were in exactly such a position, and almost all of them say that it was just a bit of a pain and that it wasn't a positive experience. In my opinion, that is not a constructive or beneficial use of your time. The CV points derived from a higher degree are a welcome bonus, but really ought not to be the primary reason to proceed.

WHAT DIFFERENT SKILLS DO YOU NEED FOR RESEARCH?

One of the best things about research is that you can learn new skills and techniques as you go, and these may be useful for the rest of your career, including during clinical training. When you are just starting out in research, it is not necessarily your skills that will bring success, but your attitude, aspirations, and enthusiasm.

Being a researcher is a bit like being an entrepreneur. You need to present yourself well to potential investors in both time and money in order to start your research (a bit like a start-up company). You then need to design and follow through with projects (just like a new business) – something that requires dedication and motivation. Potential supervisors and university lecturers/professors can detect these kinds of traits and will be much more likely to want to take you on as a student if you show them.

Research is not taught and examined in chunks like you may have experienced on your Bachelor's or Master's degree–level courses. It is much more self-directed, and your final research plans may look very different to what you started with. There will be setbacks and failures to overcome along the way. Therefore, success depends on both commitment and desire to follow through with things, as well as an ability to adapt to all the unexpected twists and turns that may lie in your path. If you have these attributes, then the skills required for research will come naturally and will develop throughout your studies.

DOES NORMAL MEDICAL TRAINING PREPARE YOU FOR RESEARCH?

Modern medical training usually concentrates on producing a competent, safe doctor who can learn and progress during their professional development. This approach tends to favour clinical practice rather than research. In fact, most doctors (including myself) probably skimmed through the parts of medical school that might be valuable for understanding research, such as statistics, epidemiology, and critical appraisal of medical literature. But doctors are usually, by their nature, constantly learning, teaching, and developing. Therefore, most doctors are already equipped with the basic tools they need for research – a basic scientific understanding of pathology, a desire to learn new things and improve practice, and a care for the outcomes of patients.

Because of these traits, doctors find themselves part of a relatively unique cohort of professionals that can usually transition to a period of time in research without too much difficulty. But as mentioned earlier, the components of motivation and ambition that got you into medical school in the first place should be revived, nurtured, and harnessed for you to approach the higher levels of uncertainty in research when compared with your clinical 'day job'.

WHAT IS ENJOYABLE AND WHAT IS CHALLENGING ABOUT RESEARCH?

The most enjoyable aspect of research for me was the independent working style that it allowed for. I shaped my working week between family activities, dedicated time for reading and writing, and laboratory experiments. This meant that on some days, I worked until late in the evening, and other days I just didn't do any work at all – and mostly on my own terms. This meant that I could be very productive and flexible at the same time.

One of the biggest challenges in research is the fact that often things don't necessarily go the way you planned. There will be times when you don't feel as if you're getting anywhere, and others when something went wrong in the laboratory, or you need to go back and get more data, or your project needs to change direction in order to produce useful data.

As a junior doctor in clinical practice, there are usually more senior doctors around who could 'rescue' a situation that wasn't going as intended (like a cannula that you can't get or a sick patient that requires a senior review). However, in your research, it is sometimes up to you to come up with a pragmatic solution for your own work. Although there are opportunities to discuss problems and plans with your supervisors, ultimately you are the one who needs to direct and initiate the subsequent plan.

My research topic (even the title, aims, and objectives) all evolved throughout my research based on what was feasible and what went well. Now that I have been through it all, I believe that it has helped my personal development in terms of problem solving and adaptation. These will hopefully be of use in the future!

HOW DO JUNIOR DOCTORS GET INVOLVED?

If you are thinking of taking some time out of training for research, the first step would be to discuss with colleagues and friends who have done some research already. You may find that every individual has had a slightly different experience and can offer a wide range of stories (both good and bad). Then the next step would be to approach a mentor or academic leader – perhaps your educational supervisor, a consultant you work with, or a university lecturer.

You don't need to have a fully formed, scientifically robust plan in your head for your research. Your ideas and plans will develop over time and will probably evolve into something completely different to what you started with. But the important thing to do is to discuss widely, and to start to establish in your mind, whether research is something you'd like to do.

During these preliminary conversations, it may also be worthwhile trying to write an article or two so that you can determine whether you enjoy that kind of thing. This might be a review article on a topic that interests you, or some research at your place of work. Again, seeking help from others that have done it before would be the most useful plan. If you do choose to take steps to apply for time out of training, you will need letters of support from your clinical and educational supervisors, potential higher-degree supervisors, and your training deanery – so the earlier you initiate this process, the better.

CASE STUDY

At a relatively early part of my surgical training, I decided to take some time out of clinical practice to do a three-year doctorate. I did this for a few reasons. Firstly, I had been working on some projects during core surgical training and started to really enjoy writing but was a bit frustrated that this kind of academic work had to be undertaken outside of normal working hours – a kind of extracurricular activity demanded by modern training. I wanted to do some more in-depth research in a full-time capacity rather than trying to fit it in around other training activities. Secondly, I wanted to spend more weekends and nights at home with my family, rather than doing shifts at the hospital. And thirdly, I felt that my longer-term career plan should involve both academic and clinical work, so I wanted to incorporate a research element into my career pathway. It was really the combination of these factors which made me finally take the plunge and pause my surgical training.

One of the projects in my research was investigating the way the microcirculation behaves after injury and haemorrhage. I used a handheld microscope to scan the microcirculation under the tongues of patients presenting to the emergency department after major trauma.

In order to do this, I had to learn how to apply for research ethics committee approval, set up a research site, and learn how to do the scanning. I also took blood samples from the patients, which I had to centrifuge and store in the laboratory. That also involved learning some new techniques (such as ELISA), which I was taught by my supervisor and laboratory staff.

I worked with my supervisors to come up with some novel research questions, then had to design the data collection tools, and then analyse the data. Again, these were techniques that I learnt along the way.

Every time we performed an analysis, we came up with even more research questions. This was an exciting journey, because we were getting results that had never been reported before, and we also had the freedom to take the research questions in whatever direction we wanted. I had the opportunity to present some of this work at various national and international conferences, and of course, published the papers that formed chapters in my thesis.

> The whole process was planned in a certain order at the start of my research, but ended up in a totally different order, with some analyses that had not been previously considered. Putting everything together in a logical order in my thesis was a really rewarding experience, since it was really the first time that everything seemed to come together and make sense!

CONCLUSION

Taking time out of clinical training to undertake some research offers an opportunity to change your style and pace of work, learn new skills and techniques, and gain an in-depth knowledge of a topic of your choice. As well as preparing you for a possible academic career, and bulking up the CV, research is a chance to have some independence in your working life and to develop and test new ideas. It isn't for everyone, and the journey can be tortuous, but if you are motivated, adaptable, enthusiastic, and follow through with plans, it may be just right for you.

7.2

Entrepreneur

LEWIS POTTER

Over the years of studying and training that it takes to become a doctor, doctors acquire a huge range of skills and a breadth of specialist knowledge that can be an underestimated personal resource. Doctors are also trained communicators and have been taught to think through and solve complex problems, so it is probably natural that many doctors have ideas which have the potential to be marketed.

Bringing ideas or products to the marketplace is not only a good way to broaden your career and experience a working world outside of healthcare, it can also be of huge benefit to our patients and to wider society.

WHY BE AN ENTREPRENEUR?

Some might argue that being a doctor or medical student is stressful enough without the added pressure of starting up a business, and in many ways, they are probably right. Your daily workload will almost certainly increase and the boundary between what is work and what is your own time will become even more blurred.

However, starting a business is an opportunity to do something completely different, to introduce variety into your work life, potentially make a difference to lots of people's lives, and possibly make money.

Starting something new and working to make it grow and flourish is enormously satisfying, and finding satisfaction in this new and different area of work can provide huge relief from the feelings of stress and burnout that are all too common in medicine.

HARNESSING EXISTING SKILLS

Doctors possess a very valuable core set of skills that are very adaptable and relevant to most businesses, within or outside of healthcare. Generally, doctors are very hardworking and understand the importance of task prioritisation and efficiency. This ability to effectively manage time is a huge asset when starting a new business, particularly if you are setting up whilst working the day job.

Doctors are lifelong learners and are used to adapting to a constantly changing environment (e.g. changing placements, changing guidelines, changing clinical scenarios). This mindset of adaptability and the willingness to learn new skills can enable any budding entrepreneur to react to the changes in their marketplace, allowing their business to grow and evolve as the situation demands. As a result of the continually changing landscape in which any new business is likely to find itself, an entrepreneur needs to be prepared to constantly make decisions, assess the impact of those decisions, and then use that as feedback to improve future decision making, a process much like the audit cycles with which we are all familiar in medicine.

Medical students and doctors have spent years learning communication skills and practicing these in the most stressful and emotionally demanding situations. This is a real asset to have as a founder, where you need to be able to communicate goals clearly, delegate appropriately to other team members, and listen carefully to feedback. There will be times when team members will have difficulties, or when you may need to let someone go from the company, both of which require you as the founder to communicate with empathy.

Clearly, it is also important to be able to communicate your company's vision to its target audience and, whilst marketing may be a less natural skill for many doctors, being able to communicate accurately, concisely, and empathetically is a skill in which we are all trained and which can be built upon.

Just as in medicine, there are few quick wins in business. Perseverance and the ability to keep working towards something, despite little to no short-term benefit, is definitely something that you need in business. The 'overnight successes' that you hear about in the start-up world are, in reality, often preceded by several years of hard work, failures, and doubt. It's the ability to take those failures, learn from them and, most importantly, not give up that is essential for starting a business. The majority of businesses fail because the founding team loses motivation and gives up.

Medics are also trained to recognise where the limits of their competence lie and to ask for help and specialist input when required. When entering the world of business, this same attitude will help ensure the safety of your investment.

LEARNING NEW SKILLS

Many doctors are naturally altruistic and find it uncomfortable to ask people to pay money for something, particularly those of us who have trained in the NHS where the idea of 'free at the point of need' underpins everything. But for a business to be successful, it needs to generate revenue to cover running costs (at the very least), so becoming better at describing the value of what you are providing and then asking for something in return is essential. These marketing skills are things that we aren't taught in medicine and so may be an area that you might need help with.

Perfectionist personality types are common amongst medical students and doctors who are used to being high achievers. To be a successful entrepreneur, you may need to resist this tendency, as it can lead to an inability to release a product or launch an idea until you feel it is 'perfect'. This approach can result in an excessive investment of time and money before the product ever sees the light of day. As a result, you end up developing a product in a vacuum, with no early feedback from the audience you are hoping to serve, until you eventually present them with your 'perfect' product. This approach significantly increases the risk of building something that nobody wants.

Alternatively, by releasing a product early, in its most basic form (often referred to as a minimally viable product or MVP), you get immediate feedback before you've invested too much time or money. You can then continue to develop the product, basing your strategic direction and feature set on real user feedback, ultimately increasing the chances that you'll achieve product–market fit (a.k.a. build something people actually want).

Depending on what type of business you are starting you may wish to seek formal training to help you along the way. There are numerous business and management qualifications that can be obtained through universities or colleges, but these can be time-consuming and costly. There are also numerous online modules to help you pick up skills in specific areas such as accounting and human resources. However, many key insights are less tangible and only become apparent through the experience of running your own business.

FINDING INSPIRATION

Wherever there are problems or inefficiencies, there is the potential to create solutions and businesses around them. The healthcare field is littered with these opportunities whether you look at medical education, the use of technology in healthcare, system structure, or direct patient care.

Really, it's a question of finding a problem or inefficiency that you're passionate about improving. Passion about the problem is essential, because that's the only thing you'll have to motivate you through the difficult times of running your own business.

FINDING HELP

There are so many resources available to help people who want to get started with building a company that it's actually quite difficult to pick just a few to discuss here. Google searches such as 'how to start a business' or 'how to launch a product' will deliver a plethora of websites, blogs, and companies all eager to offer advice and guidance. As ever, approach online resources with a touch of scepticism and caution and try to find reputable sources of help.

One incredibly invaluable resource which has been designed specifically to help medics is the Clinical Entrepreneur Training Program, which has been created by NHS England to support clinical staff who want to work on an entrepreneurial project alongside training.[1] The program provides educational events that cover key topics relevant to all businesses, such as how to build a team, how to develop an initial product, and how to iterate based on feedback. It also provides a great network of like-minded clinicians and mentors who have lots of previous experience to help you along your journey.

Another very useful resource that I've found really valuable is Y Combinator's Startup School, which is a series of lectures from seasoned entrepreneurs on how to start a company (free videos available online).[2]

PITFALLS

Starting a business will never be without risk and sacrifice, and it is not always possible to know what the scale of those risks and sacrifices will be until you are already well underway.

The major pitfall, particularly at the start, will be a loss of work–life balance. You are potentially taking on another full-time job to fit in around an already busy work life, and you may quickly see evenings and weekends vanish.

The second major pitfall is financial over-commitment. Many ideas can be developed relatively cheaply, but others will require investment, which may come from personal savings, external investors, or bank loans. In an ideal world, you would only invest what you can safely afford to lose, but it may be that you need to seek extra funds from elsewhere. If this is the case, make sure your borrowing is based on sound planning rather than gut instinct, and try to have an exit strategy if things are not going well. Taking financial advice from the business advisors at your bank is a sensible place to start if looking for extra money to invest.

If your business is successful, you may find it difficult to keep up with the demands of your training program, and you may need to accept that you need to extend your training either by taking time out or going part time.

CASE STUDY

I started Geeky Medics whilst I was a fourth-year medical student at Newcastle University. I was fascinated by the internet's growing potential and simultaneously disappointed by the lack of online medical education that was freely accessible. As a result, I launched the Geeky Medics website (after several months of trial and error and annoying people much more technical than me on various online forums).

I started to share my own notes on the website and then convinced some friends to feature in clinical skills videos which we published online. As I continued to work on the site, the number of views slowly increased and our audience grew, presumably through word of mouth. It's now almost eight years later and we receive over two million views of our content every month from a global audience of medical students and other healthcare professionals.

Geeky Medics adds a lot of variety to my week around the clinical commitments of GP training. It certainly can be stressful at times, but it does mean I never find myself bored or stuck in the same old routine. The days working on Geeky Medics can be incredibly varied, including strategic planning, content production, discussions with the YouTube team, replying to medical students all over the world and updating our mobile apps. My days working as a GP trainee offer a similarly broad variety of presentations, so I feel like I'm constantly learning and broadening my understanding.

As much as I love working on Geeky Medics, it does present several challenges, particularly making it work alongside training. I can't say how much time I've invested in Geeky Medics over the last eight years, but I know it's a lot, and there have been times, such as during foundation training, when it was incredibly difficult to keep working on the project.

I'm now a part-time (60%) GP trainee, meaning I have two days a week dedicated to managing the project. This still isn't enough to feel on top of all elements of the business, but it's a lot better than my previous experience when I was a full-time trainee. Historically, I have been responsible for almost every task within the project, from content production, filming, video editing, website maintenance, graphic design, marketing, accounting, customer support, and hiring. As a result, I work most evenings after clinical work on the project and at least one day each weekend (but often both). I try to prioritise as best as I can, but the feeling of continually spinning plates is at times incredibly stressful. You can probably guess that my work–life balance isn't great, and I'm working on improving it through building a team and getting better at delegating tasks to those who can do a much better job than me.

As a result of working part-time on Geeky Medics, my GP training will take longer (five years instead of three). I make sure to prioritise things like portfolio and extracurricular learning above the project's needs (which can feel difficult at times).

I've tried my best to avoid financial risk with the project by only investing in expansion when there is a clear demand from the user base. I have no external investors, so I've had the luxury of choosing a safe pace for the project to scale at.

I run Geeky Medics as a social enterprise (broadly speaking, this is a business that seeks to maximise its positive social impact). Geeky Medics is a combination of all of my interests, including connected technologies, video production, graphic design, and my passion for medical education. As a result, I genuinely love working on the project, and the community that has grown around Geeky Medics helps motivate me to keep pushing forward.

CONCLUSION

Doctors and medical students are intelligent, highly educated, and motivated people and, as such, are ideally suited to entrepreneurship. Medics often underestimate their own value and that of their creations, but by having the confidence to take their ideas to the marketplace they can add enormous value to their own careers and to the wider world of healthcare.

REFERENCES

1. Clinical Entrepreneurs Training Programme. Available: www.england.nhs.uk, search on 'clinical entrepreneurs'. Accessed: 19th August 2018.
2. Startup School, Available: www.startupschool.org. Accessed: 19th August 2018.

7.3

Medical writer

ADAM STATEN

Medicine is endlessly intriguing both for those involved with providing care to patients and for lay people. For those who like to write, inspiration can be found everywhere in our working lives, whether you want to write about the way care is delivered, new and innovative treatments, or, perhaps more philosophically, the way that people interact at times of high stress and emotion. Well-written work on any of these topics will never lack for an audience, and as a doctor or medical student, we have privileged access to expert knowledge and to rare experiences that can provide fascinating subject matter.

There are also more platforms than ever before on which to write and get a message out to a wider audience, and writing can provide an outlet for frustrations and a way to instigate change. It is also a way to engage with people, share ideas, learn, and educate.

WHY WRITE?

Every day we are exposed to complex and emotionally provoking situations which may leave us at a loss for a way forward or may inspire within us an idea for how things can be done better. However we are left feeling, writing can provide a way for us to share the experience and spark a debate that may provide the solution we seek, or propagate and develop the ideas we have had.

Medicine is a collaboration, and writing provides a means for us to collaborate with more people than those immediately around us and to collaborate with people in different industries or the wider public in general. It is a way to share the lessons learned across the world so that we can improve the way we care for our patients.

Also, and perhaps more importantly in terms of avoiding burnout, writing can be an incredibly cathartic process. Life as a doctor can be very frustrating, and these frustrations have a tendency to fester if left unvented. Writing is a way to air these frustrations and, more often than not, a way to find that there are others who share them and may have an answer to them. It is a constructive way to address the numerous inaccuracies and falsehoods about healthcare that are spread via both the mainstream media and social media.

Writing can also be a boost for your CV. It is a way of showing that you engage with current thinking within medicine and that you have your own thoughts on the subject. This can make you stand out above your peers whether your publications are well grounded in research or whether they are opinion pieces that show that you are someone with your own mind. Whilst a blog or a magazine article might just add colour to your CV, a letter to a journal will gain you a cheap citable reference, and a published paper will add meaningfully to the literature.

Sadly, medical writing is unlikely to make you rich, but there are opportunities to pick up some extra cash by writing. The knowledge we all possess is hard-earned and valuable and of huge interest to people the world over. If you are able to make medical topics accessible and understandable, then that is a marketable gift. Money can be earned writing content for websites, editing translations of academic publications from other countries, writing patient information literature for industries such as pharmaceuticals, or even writing commissioned books designed with a particular (usually fairly niche) audience in mind.

Work such as this can be found on freelancing websites such as upwork.com or the European Medical Writers Association website. Be warned though, competition can be fierce as there are plenty of people who like to write, so this is very much a buyer's market.

Above all, writing is enjoyable. Being able to put your thoughts into words and knowing that others are reading them, and hopefully paying attention to them, can be both exciting and satisfying. If life in the day job can be very stressful, having something enjoyable and mentally engaging to do in your time off can go a long way to stopping that stress from becoming all-consuming.

With sharing on social media, your message can go from your mind to a worldwide audience of tens of thousands within a few minutes, and this can feel empowering in a way that few of us get to experience whilst walking the wards.

GETTING STARTED

When it comes to getting things published, there is something of a paradox: editors and publishers are often only interested in those with a proven track record, but it is impossible to develop a track record if no one will publish you. As someone with no writing experience, it will be very difficult to go straight to getting regular work writing for a mainstream publication, or a big medical journal, or even getting a book published no matter how great your ideas are.

The key is to start small and to write frequently. Platforms on which to write are everywhere. Online publications are usually the easiest to break into, and lots of medical institutions (hospitals, medical schools, campaign groups, and charities) have blogs that welcome contributions. Blogs often publish articles very frequently in order to keep their presence felt and their profile high, and they therefore need a high volume of contributions. Blogs are also readily shared and give the writer the opportunity to interact with his or her audience, which can raise a writer's profile very quickly.

Similarly, letters to journals, newspapers, and magazines have much less stringent editorial criteria than full articles but will add to your writing portfolio. Health websites are in abundance and all need content, so if you are happy to write about the health benefits of the Mediterranean diet or ten ways to avoid diabetes, you can often find a website who will publish it for you.

A portfolio of articles and publications, even if they are on relatively obscure platforms, shows editors that you are someone who can write, and this makes you a much more attractive prospect.

Don't underestimate the importance of social media. Sharing via Facebook, Twitter, or other social media sites can hugely increase your reach, and if you can build up a social media following, then this will appeal to editors who will see that, by using you, they are also gaining access to the people who follow you.

PITCHING YOUR WORK

Whenever you are pitching a piece or an idea to a publication, it is important to pay attention to three things: who their audience is, what style of work they like to publish, and what their submission guidelines are. If you misjudge or ignore any one of these three things, then you are completely wasting your time by contacting them.

The audience of the publication will very much reflect the agenda of the publication – and they all have an agenda. This agenda may be obvious, for example it is safe to assume that a cardiology journal is interested in disseminating new knowledge about subjects relevant to keeping people's hearts healthy, but mainstream media publications are likely to have a social and political agenda. For example, there is no point sending an article about the merits of private healthcare to a left-leaning newspaper such as *The Guardian*.

Styles vary considerably too. An academic publication is likely to be formal in style, with an expectation that arguments will be balanced and well-evidenced, but a blog will expect its authors to write pieces that fuel debate and perhaps court controversy. Read examples of things they have previously published; see what language is used. Is this intended for a lay or a healthcare-professional audience? If it is for a lay audience, is it for young mums or ageing bachelors? The style of the publication will also dictate the length of the articles they publish. Blog posts, for example, tend to be around 600 words in length because readers start switching off once they hit around 1000 words. This is a tight limit in which to say everything you may wish to say, so your writing will need to be concise and punchy and this may only be possible by sacrificing balance.

Most publications have submission guidelines on their websites. Follow them to the letter if you expect anyone to read your work. Editors receive a lot of submissions and the first to be discarded are from the writers who don't bother to follow the rules.

COMMON PITFALLS

Writing is a fairly low-risk activity compared with the things that we do in our day jobs, but it is not completely without risk.

Most importantly, never ever use patient identifiable information unless you have cast iron consent from a patient to do so. This is a very quick way to sink a budding medical career. You may think that no one will recognise the photo of that groin rash but the patient will and may be very unhappy to find out that you've used it.

Try not to be rude and offensive. This can be difficult once people have started responding to an article you have written, particularly because they may be rude, offensive, and ignorant themselves. Just remember that what you write is out in the world forever and may come back to haunt you in years to come. The momentary satisfaction of putting an ignoramus back in their box may pale to insignificance when those comments are quoted back to you at some unforeseen future date.

Be careful not to quote erroneous or fabricated data. When writing for a mainstream or lay publication it is tempting not to hold yourself to the rigour expected in academic publications. Wherever you are writing, remember that you are still writing as a medical professional. Whilst the length of an article may not allow you to do full justice to all the available evidence, ensure that the evidence you do use is reliable and accurate.

CASE STUDY

I had never really thought about medical writing, but a few years ago there was a widely publicised medical story that was covered with varying degrees of hysteria and medical illiteracy by almost all mainstream media outlets. The details of the case weren't particularly of concern to me but I was upset by the implicit criticism of the NHS and its staff that came across in almost every discussion of it. In something of a fit of pique, I wrote a letter to a national newspaper about how the morale of those of us working in the NHS was being crushed by the continual pernicious criticism exemplified by this case. I was shocked when it got published, but it was an incredible buzz to see my thoughts out there for all to read, and more so when response letters of support were published the following week.

At the time, I was a GP trainee and, with the wind in my sails, I started writing articles that I thought might be of interest to the readers of the *British Journal of General Practice*. Luckily for me, the journal was just then setting up its blog, and the editorial team was looking for people who could turn out regular pieces to get the blog going. As with many blogs, particularly in the start-up phase, they were keen for pieces that would raise its profile and get conversations going. With this in mind, I wrote a few tongue-in-cheek pieces (for example how a particular item of clothing was a red-flag sign of psychosocial distress), which I very much doubt the blog or journal would now publish.

This opened my eyes to a world of blogging, and now, with a few articles and blog posts in my back pocket, I started blogging on more mainstream sites such as the *Huffington Post*. At the same time, I found that I could make a little pocket money writing articles for websites (things such as '10 ways to lower your blood pressure without medication' and 'the myths and facts about weight loss'), and I spent some time editing academic papers that had been translated from Polish.

As a result of this, I was asked to contribute a chapter about blogging and writing to a book aimed at medical students. The author/editor of that book sent me his own chapter 'how to get a book published' as an example of what he wanted, which I read with great interest. A few years later, and I now have two books of my own published and I have also edited a major medical textbook. This has often been hard work, and has definitely required a significant time commitment with very little financial reward, but it has provided variety in my work and quite a lot of personal satisfaction.

CONCLUSION

There are numerous reasons to write, and there are numerous opportunities to do so. Whether your motivation is personal, academic, political, social, or financial, sharing your thoughts and ideas is a fantastic way to contribute to the collaborative endeavour that is healthcare. It may require perseverance but can ultimately be enormously satisfying.

7.4

Manager

MARTIN McSHANE

Worldwide health systems are facing immense challenges. To some extent, we are victims of huge success! People are living longer. We can do more with diagnostics and treatments. We are on the verge of a new era driven by our understanding of genomics. I strongly believe the medical profession has a vital role to play in shaping and delivering twenty-first century health and care. We can do that on a one-to-one basis. In fact, we must continue to do that on a one-to-one basis. However, there is good evidence that where doctors step into the space of system management, they can make an important contribution to not only delivering the triple aim of better experience and outcomes for patients with better use of resources, but also to deliver a fourth aim – joy in work for professionals.

As a former surgeon and director of clinical governance for the NHS, Aidan Halligan said in 2006, 'We need to move from a culture of performance management to one of performance leadership … The healthcare system is populated by bright, dedicated, well intentioned people. Now is the time to surface that talent in meaningful leadership positions across the NHS and, together with smart processes and enabling technology, allow the best mediocre healthcare service in the world to become truly the very best'.

WHY?

Simon Sinek, an organizational consultant, once gave a great talk in which he reflects on what drives purpose – the 'why'? Surfacing what drives you is helpful in making career choices. For me, leaving surgical training and retraining and working in General Practice (GP) was a salutary experience. Firstly, working in the acute sector had me utterly unprepared for the challenges of the specialism of General Practice. I believe that General Practice is the most difficult specialty to excel at. It perfectly encompasses Osler's dictum, 'Medicine is a science of uncertainty and an art of probability'.

The implementation of GP fundholding (a scheme in the 1990s in which GPs held budgets with which to purchase or commission services for their patients) taught me about pragmatism and helped me understand the importance of the triple aim. As I started as a partner, my practice which was politically, philosophically, and practically opposed to fundholding suddenly changed its position. Why? Because through fundholding, we could improve patient care. A core value for the partnership was high-quality care. Looking at the information on activity and funding made us realise we were not delivering the best experience, outcomes, or use of resources for the population we served. In essence, fundholding was my first exposure to population health management.

By grappling with the available data, we found we could significantly improve multiple aspects of the care we wanted to provide and make better use of the resources available. Not only did that align with the triple aim, but also it improved our own professional experience (delivering the 'quadruple aim').

As I became more and more engaged with understanding how the system worked, I began to realise how important it was for doctors to become involved in the governance, design, and implementation of that system. At the heart of this is an essential belief that the vast majority of professionals (doctors, nurses, pharmacists, allied health professionals, social workers) get up every day with the intent of doing their best. It is not the individuals that fail, but the system that fails them. A pivotal moment for me was when the vice chancellor of a university came to speak to a learning set of GPs just before the introduction of Primary Care Groups (effectively the next iteration of fundholding). He challenged us: 'you can either sit and moan about your lot or you can roll your sleeves up and get involved in shaping how the future works'. At its simplest, that is why I transitioned into management.

CAPABILITIES

It is unlikely that doctors will lack the intellect for a role in management. However, in itself, intellect is desirable but insufficient. Having a brain the size of a planet is inadequate without the right atmosphere around it to sustain life. Medicine is a human endeavour, based on humane values and is about human beings. It requires emotional intelligence. Emotional intelligence combined with a rigorous intellect, whenever I have encountered it, has been a terrific force for good. Daniel Goleman raised awareness of emotional intelligence some twenty years ago.[1] He now describes four essential components:

1. Self-awareness
2. Self-management
3. Social awareness
4. Relationship management

It is not difficult to describe, but practising all four, especially in pressurised and stressful circumstances, is not always easy.

Based on personal experience, if I were to choose one core skill which amplifies emotional intelligence, it would be to study and practice coaching. It is not the only skill you will need, but I would propose it as the most important.

A very good CEO I worked for asked me, in an early one-to-one, how many management styles I had and which I favoured. The essence of this question, I believe, is exploring whether you need to be directive, facilitative, mentoring, or coaching as a manager. The right answer is all four are necessary and depend on the context. The skill is to know when to use which style. There are times when it is essential to be directive, but your job will be easier and your team function much better if you use a coaching style which makes the most of an individual's and a team's potential.

Any doctor moving into management will need to learn about and value some practical skills in the same way we do for medicine. Moreover, many of these capabilities are inherently of value in the practice of medicine. I sometimes wish that I had some of the training earlier from which I benefited in the latter half of my career. Time management, chairing meetings, programme and project management, facilitation, and coaching skills have all been beneficial to me.

Some skills are more difficult to acquire and develop. A good example, for me, is a definition of wisdom I recently heard as being the ability to choose the right gap between stimulus and response. The best clinicians and managers I have worked with have been masters of judging that timing. Sometimes it has to be short, an instinctive reaction, and sometimes real wisdom is knowing when not to make a decision until a decision has to be made.

A final capability, which I believe is perhaps one of the most important for both the professions of medicine and management, is resilience. A mentor and friend said to me, 'As you become more senior in management the more you will need to draw upon the well of resource that is inside you'. An article which I recommend to colleagues, who are working in pressurised circumstances, is 'Manage your energy, not your time'.[2] Consciously paying attention to the four aspects of physical, emotional, psychological, and spiritual energy has been helpful for me on my career journey. I would add that some of that has been a retrospective realisation that luckily or instinctively I was doing the right things, but they have been complemented by active contemplation of what more I could do to help myself, my colleagues, and my family.

TRAINING AND DEVELOPMENT

As a medical student, surgical trainee, and general practitioner, I have benefited from a well-trodden path for clinicians of training and skills acquisition. The latter half of my career has been littered with a far less structured but very rich and varied array of training opportunities.

Let me start, however, with some research that I first heard presented at an NHS Confederation conference.[3] The research examined whether people were lucky or not. The answer seemed to be that some were. Why? Fundamentally, it seemed to be because they were open to opportunity. They made themselves aware of it. The point of this story is that opportunity for training abounds. The art is in being receptive and willing to take advantage of it. So, what is out there?

Courses

Many doctors entering into management undertake an MBA (Master of Business Administration), which can be studied at numerous universities around the country or by distance learning. This can be costly (up to tens of thousands of pounds at some top institutions) but can give you a firm grounding in understanding how businesses run (including those involved with healthcare).

The New York–based Commonwealth Fund runs Harkness Fellowships in which fellows spend 12 months in the United States, conducting original research and working with leading US health-policy experts. Having met a number of participants over the years, it would seem to be an invaluable experience.

I am deeply envious of colleagues who have been on the Institute for Healthcare Improvement (IHI) Fellowship programme. Fellows spend a year immersing themselves in learning about healthcare improvement. With funding from the family of George W. Merck, the Health Foundation (UK), and Kaiser Permanente, the fellows plunge into projects, gain technical improvement skills, meet the world's foremost improvement leaders, and tour innovative healthcare systems. When they return home, they often take on new leadership roles at work.

Here in the UK, two organisations are a rich resource of opportunity. Firstly there is the NHS Leadership Academy, which offers a rich and varied set of programmes from first steps to supporting people who aspire to CEO roles. Secondly, and aimed specifically at doctors, is the Faculty of Medical Leadership and Management. As a resource and portal for the needs of doctors interested in management, I would strongly recommend becoming a member. It coordinates the National Clinical Fellow scheme, which is a great opportunity for junior doctors to get exposure to senior leaders in the NHS and private sector and gain insights into system management that few other schemes provide.

There are numerous programmes to support people in developing coaching skills. I obtained a PgC from Teesside University, but geography may dictate the location of such a course for an individual, and careful research will find the right one for you. There are also numerous one-, two-, or three-day courses on which to develop skills across the spectrum of skills that will be required of you as a manager.

Structured learning from courses, such as those described above, is helpful. However, it is only a small component of the time one spends learning. A colleague from Health Education England framed it for me like this: 'About 5% of learning comes from structured courses, 10% from self-directed learning and the rest is experiential – learning on the job'. I grew up in an era when one had to lug textbooks around and access research through journals. The cornucopia of material now available and different ways of accessing it leaves no excuse for a lack of materials for self-directed learning. Increasingly, the art is learning how to navigate it all!

CASE STUDY

As a medical student, I was in a tutorial with a professor of surgery during my final year. He asked us why we had come to medical school. We said, 'to learn medicine'; he replied, 'you are here to pass finals, you will be learning about medicine for the next 40 years'.

Nearly 40 years later, I realise how right he was. I am still learning and have had a rich and varied career through training in surgery; being a GP partner; into local, regional, and national roles in NHS commissioning; and now working in the private sector. The wonderful thing about a medical degree is the rich portfolio career it offers. There is no need to be bored or burnt out: you can find ways to be challenged, stretched, and rewarded in so many different ways. Would I change the career path I have followed? No. Would I do it all over again? Instantly. Has it all been fun and enjoyable? No, certainly not. There have been times of deep dismay (and tears). It is the contrasts, however, that have made it so fulfilling and rewarding. This case study, I hope, illustrates this.

Only two years after leaving my practice I faced the fact that the primary care trust (PCT) I was CEO for was being merged. I had to seek a new job. I could have gone back into practice but chose to apply and become an executive director in a very large PCT. With a budget of a billion pounds for a population of 750 thousand people, I had an immediate task to engage the local people, politicians, and professionals in accepting some significant changes. Supported by a terrific board, CEO, and executive colleagues, I worked closely with an immensely skilled manager.

This dyad of clinician and manager working in partnership has always, in my experience, been much greater than the sum of its parts. Engaging and supporting local clinicians, working with the public, and using data and professional expertise, we were able to secure overwhelming support to close an A&E and change the use of a much-loved, but small and isolated, hospital from traditional ways of working into a new care model. This also avoided closing down a unit which brought much economic benefit to the local community — something not often considered when reconfiguring services.

As a doctor, you can and will help many individuals. By stepping into the space offered by system management, you can contribute to helping many thousands of people. Having had the opportunity, I can thoroughly recommend a career which embraces both.

CONCLUSION

I have had a wonderful career and been exposed to rich and varied experiences. The privilege of being a doctor is something I treasure. Being invited into other people's lives, to hopefully help them but always care for them, should never be taken for granted. To do that in the most effective way requires doctors to also immerse themselves in the complexity and challenges of designing and implementing the systems and processes that support all professionals in that endeavour. That, to me, is why some of us need to take our knowledge and experience of patient care and help lead and manage the health and care system.

REFERENCES

1. Goleman D. 1995. *Emotional Intelligence*. New York: Bantam Books.
2. Schwartz T, McCarthy, C. Manage Your Energy, Not Your Time. Harvard Business Review, October 2007.
3. Wiseman R. May 2003. The luck factor. *Skeptical Inquirer* 27(3).

RECOMMENDED READING

I will keep this to a short selection of the books (and articles) that I feel have had the biggest influence on my thinking and behaviours and which I hope will be useful to any doctor considering taking on a management role.

Scholte P. 1997. *The Leader's Handbook*. McGraw Hill Professional.

Gawande A. 2014. *Being Mortal: Illness, Medicine and What Matters in the End*. London: Wellcome Collection.

Harford T. 2011. *Adapt: Why Success Always Starts With Failure*. London: Hachette Digital.

Whitmore J. 2009. *Coaching for Performance*. London: Hodder and Stoughton.

McChrystal GS. 2015. *Team of Teams*. Portfolio Penguin.

7.5

Military doctor

MAX MARSDEN

Being in the military can be tough both physically and mentally; it's not for everyone. For those that crave to perform 'good medicine in bad places', it's the opportunity of a lifetime. The British Military exists to protect the UK, prevent conflict, deal with disaster, and fight the nation's enemies. If you would like a medical career supporting these objectives, the life of a military doctor could be for you.

Military doctors come in several flavours. The UK has three services that employ doctors: the Army, Navy, and Royal Air Force. Broadly, doctors in the military are either regulars (full time) or reservists (part time). The military also employs civilians to work as general practitioners (GPs) in the home base who don't deploy and won't be discussed in any more detail here. This section is about a deployable career in the military. Deployable doctors 'sign up' to work within military units and physically accompany the soldiers, sailors, and airmen of the UK military.

WHAT IS DIFFERENT ABOUT MILITARY MEDICINE AND BEING A DOCTOR IN THE MILITARY?

Military doctors are present wherever the military is deployed. The Defence Medical Services provide medical support to operations, exercises, and adventurous training all over the world. In these varied locations, military medicine ranges from providing risk assessments and casualty evacuation plans to providing immediate pre-hospital trauma care. Of course, there is also the need for hospital medicine and long-term rehabilitation, similar to the NHS, but often this medicine is provided in a very different context. For example, on recent humanitarian assistance deployments, hospital medicine has been performed at sea and under tents. This requires doctors to be robust and able to work in resource-limited environments. Military doctors treat people in need and do not only provide care for members of the Armed Forces but also their families and often civilians.

HOW DO YOU 'GET IN'?

Applications to become a regular or reserve doctor are made directly to the single service you want to join. The application process is similar between all three services, and applications are accepted at several stages during your medical career. There are medical bursaries or cadetships available to medical students within their last three years of medical school. Potential cadets are encouraged to join the Officers' Training Corps during medical school, but there is no obligation for this. Applications are also invited during foundation years or as a fully qualified consultant or GP. Applications at other times in your career (e.g. registrar training) are occasionally accepted after discussion with the specific service.

The Ministry of Defence (MOD) is a modern and inclusive organisation. But it is allowed to be selective about whom it employs. For example, there are several health conditions that preclude you from joining the military. This is because there are times in a military career when it won't be easy to get hold of medication, so even illnesses that are well-controlled and don't affect everyday life, such as well-controlled asthma, can mean that you're not eligible to join. More information about the medical standards is available here: https://apply.army.mod.uk/how-to-join/can-i-join/medical.

Providing an applicant passes the medical requirements, their suitability to be commissioned into their chosen service (Army,

Navy, or Royal Air Force (RAF)) is tested. Each service has slightly different requirements and emphasis. All require a basic level of physical fitness, some knowledge about the individual service, and evidence of leadership skills. Applicants are assessed for these qualities at a selection board which involves an interview and aptitude tests.

WHAT IS THE CAREER PATH IF YOU JOIN UP AS A REGULAR?

Depending when you join and how much the military has invested in your training, you will be required to give back a 'return of service'. Joining during medical school on one of the Medical Cadetships or Bursaries has traditionally required a six- to seven-year return of service. This is in return for the funding the military has invested in your training. Joining later in your career may have a shorter return of service attached to it.

Once a military doctor has graduated from medical school, they enter into their Foundation Programme training like any other NHS doctor. Military doctors are encouraged to work in one of the several Defence Medical Group hospitals in England. These are hospitals with a military presence, where military health practitioners work alongside their NHS colleagues. These hospitals are Frimley Park, Queen Elizabeth in Birmingham, Derriford, Northallerton, and Princess Alexandra in Portsmouth. After two years of the Foundation Programme, military doctors will leave training and enter into military training within their single service. For the Army, this starts at Sandhurst; the Navy is at Dartmouth and the RAF at Cranwell.

Now, the difference between each service becomes more pronounced. Army doctors spend two or three years of 'general duties' where they can expect to join a regiment and potentially deploy on operations or exercises. The Navy have a similar period of time in which they chose to join the surface fleet, Royal Marines, or work under the water in submarines. Finally, the RAF spend one year of general duties and then enter back into specialist training. The military training starts during this period and includes leadership training, weapons handling, physical training, and military knowledge. Marching (drill) and ironing also feature here! After the military training, doctors go onto military medical training which is bespoke to their service. In the Army, this training leads to a diploma in the Medical Care of Catastrophes.

After all this training, you go on to join an operational unit. These years out of training are a fantastic opportunity to practice medicine in a different environment. The medicine can be challenging, and skills have to be developed that an NHS career may not require. For example, you may end up as the only doctor supporting 150 soldiers in a remote operating base or as a ship's doctor on patrol in the Mediterranean for three months or on a large medical exercise to Kenya.

Once those years are over, it's on to higher medical training. The requirements to progress medically in the military are the same as those in the NHS. Military doctors take the same exams and sit the same interviews. Medical training as a regular military doctor happens within the NHS. Military trainees are looked after by the military deanery and compete for places for higher training within the military deanery but may train in most places in the country.

WHAT CAREER OPPORTUNITIES ARE THERE IN THE MILITARY?

The military employs many different types of doctor, but not quite all specialities are represented. The different services have slightly different requirements. For example, the RAF have a large aeromedical evacuation role and so require more anaesthetists than surgeons. All the services need deployable GPs and core secondary care specialties such as emergency medicine and surgeons. Other secondary care specialities that are needed in a conflict like anaesthetists and acute medics are employed by the military. Careers such as public health and occupational medicine are also offered. However, specialities such as paediatrics, care of the elderly, or obstetrics and gynaecology are rarely employed as regulars. The reserves have less restrictions about when you can join and what speciality you can practise.

WHAT OTHER OPPORTUNITIES ARE THERE IN THE MILITARY?

There are lots of opportunities in the military for adventurous training, going on expeditions, and playing sport at any level from beginner to international. All of these are actively encouraged. Medical training is of course the highest priority and many training courses and exams can be funded by the military deanery. The military deanery may also offer to pay for courses not usually available to NHS doctors, such as dive medicine or mountain medicine. There are funds available for training not directly related to your medical progression as well.

ARE THERE ANY DRAWBACKS?

There are aspects to military life that might not be acceptable to everyone. There is a need to spend time away from home and loved ones. A long deployment could see you away for six months. Deployments as a consultant are usually only three months, and whilst much of this time away from home comes with warning, some deployments can spring up at short notice. The other potential limitation with military medicine is choosing a career which is either oversubscribed within the military or not available, in which case there are typically two options open to you: either you leave the military or choose a different career in order to stay in.

CAN YOU DO IT PART TIME?

Joining the reserve is an option for all three services. It offers a variety of clinical and non-clinical experience not available in normal NHS life. The Army's reserve is split into geographically located field hospitals and nationally recruited specialist units such as the medical evacuation squadron. The Navy and RAF have similar organisations. Reservists are entitled to most of the same opportunities to play sport, access adventurous training, and receive funding for medical training. The reserve is more flexible than the regulars in terms of continuing your NHS medical practice/training where you want to be.

Deployment in the reserve is often restricted to consultants and can be on a voluntary basis. Once deployed, there is no difference in operational role between reserve and regular military doctors. A reservist will function in exactly the same way as a regular military doctor and will be required to undertake the same pre-deployment training and pass the same assessments and validations as their regular counterparts.

In the Army, joining the reserve is open to medical students, although you can't commission (become an officer) until your third year. This means spending some time as a non-commissioned officer (NCO) or private soldier, which is good for some experience. When eligible to commission, there is a requirement to complete two weeks of basic soldier training and two weeks of officer training at Sandhurst. Typically, doctors in the Army Reserve will be attached to one of the regional field hospitals, all of which deployed in various capacities during the conflict in Afghanistan. There is also the opportunity to join specialist units such as 144 (parachute regiment), 335 Medical Evacuation Regiment (335 MER), and 306 Hospital Support Regiment (306 HSR). Nationally recruited units such as 335 MER and 306 HSR have a reduced annual commitment of 19 days per year, which must include 15 days of continuous training. Regional units require a commitment of 30 days of training per year.

Pay in the Reserves is based on a daily rate, although there is an additional tax-free bounty each year if the training requirements are met. Time to complete this training requirement is increasingly supported by employers. A strength of being a reservist is the ability to maintain a flexible commitment to the forces, whilst maintaining some independence. Disadvantages include some difficulty in access to courses in competition with regular colleagues.

CASE STUDY

I joined the Army during my third year at medical school. I think everyone's motivation to join as a military medic is slightly different. For me, I had always wanted to be a doctor, but at school I really enjoyed the challenge that I got from the combined cadet force. I thought that joining the military would push me both as a person and in my medical skills. At the time I was going through the selection, I really wanted to go and provide humanitarian medical support, and I realised a lifetime career of medicine in the NHS wasn't for me.

I got a Medical Cadetship in 2005 and graduated from medical school in 2008. In my final year of medical school, I went on a military-funded medical elective to the trauma service at MedSTAR in Washington, DC. This was an amazing opportunity to see and be involved in world-class trauma care. After I graduated, I joined one of the Military Defence Hospital Units for my two Foundation Years. At that time, there were a group of about six of us that lived together in the officers' mess and worked together in the hospital. It was a fantastic introduction to being a doctor. After FY2, we went to the Royal Military Academy at Sandhurst for the Professionally Qualified Officers course. This was a 10-week, military-training course. It was a fantastic change from two years of medicine. We learnt the absolute basics of soldiering, and I left there with a huge amount of respect for the officers who remain there for a full year of training. After Sandhurst, we went on to the six-month Post Graduate Medical Officers course. This is essentially medical school for the Army, and off the back of that course, I got a Diploma in the Medical Care of Catastrophes. I left those courses as a newly minted General Duties Medical Officer, and I was posted to the Household Cavalry Regiment and 4 Medical Regiment.

Over the next two years, I went on a large armoured exercise to Canada, played sport in Australia and New Zealand, and deployed to Afghanistan for six months. In Afghanistan, I spent the majority of my time with the Kings Royal Hussars in small patrol bases near the banks of the River Helmand. I was responsible for the care of both combatants and critically injured local civilians.

When I got back from the tour, I started surgical training, and after a year of registrar training in general surgery, I was given time out of programme to complete research towards a PhD. My research is about helping to improve decision making for medics treating trauma patients with machine learning tools. I am supervised by both a military and civilian academic. Without the military's advice and encouragement, I do not think I would have ever seen research as part of my career. When I finish the PhD next year, I will go back into training, and I hope to do a fellowship in trauma surgery near the end of my training. With a little luck, I hope to get a consultant job in a major trauma centre and deploy overseas again. I hope one day to deploy on a humanitarian mission, as that was my driving motivation to join 15 years ago.

CONCLUSION

Life as a military doctor opens up a world of new opportunities and experiences but it's not for everyone. The required qualities include being mentally and physically robust. Courage, leadership, initiative, and discipline are desirable. There is no getting around the fact that being in the military narrows not only the type of doctor you can be but also the places you can work, but if you're willing to be flexible, a full and professionally rewarding career is on offer.

7.6

Overseas doctor

MIKE FORSYTHE

Foundation doctors are leaving NHS training in droves, on a temporary basis at least.

In 2017, only 55% of FY2 doctors chose to apply for specialty training,[1] down from over 70% in 2011.[2] Doctors at every stage of training choose to take time out and work overseas, but many see the end of foundation training in particular as a natural opportunity to try something new.

Many of those choosing not to progress will have chosen to work abroad, but the absolute numbers of those moving overseas for work is difficult to accurately calculate. All of those taking the plunge and applying for jobs in other countries require a Certificate of Current Professional Status from the GMC, and although there are other reasons for applying for this document, the number of applications gives some indication as to the number of doctors seeking to work abroad. In 2016, certificates were issued to almost 5000 doctors in the UK.[3] Almost half of those were for Australia and New Zealand, but certificates were requested for a multitude of countries, from Afghanistan to Zimbabwe.

REASONS FOR WORKING ABROAD

Despite the threat of financial penalties for those choosing to leave the country in search of work,[4] the option to take time out of the

NHS to seek employment in hospitals and GP surgeries overseas has remained a popular one. Reasons cited in a study of FY2 doctors in Scotland included easy availability of jobs overseas, greater respect afforded to the position of a doctor in other countries, and a negative view of the NHS as a whole.[5]

Certainly, many feel a sense of disillusionment about working in healthcare in the UK, a feeling no doubt perpetuated by the standoff between the government and the BMA over the Junior Doctors contract. Many find the NHS overly bureaucratic, particularly when it comes to the process of revalidation, or are put off by exorbitant indemnity fees.[6]

Some simply feel as though they need a change of scenery, or are not yet ready to commit their professional lives to a particular specialty. Others view jobs abroad as an opportunity or a challenge. Medicine is a hugely transferable skill, and one that will never be lacking in demand. There is a chance to work in countries where the healthcare system is largely similar to the NHS, such as Australia and New Zealand, or to try something completely different, working in countries with rudimentary healthcare or limited resources.

For those seeking it, there are financial rewards available overseas. Both consultant and GP salaries in countries such as the US and Australia compare favourably to their UK counterparts. In Australia, there are financial incentives for working overtime, and it is possible to claim a proportion of every salary tax-free, further boosting one's earning potential. Actual working hours are shorter in Australia, too. Most hospital junior doctors are contracted to work a 40-hour week as opposed to the 48 hours of an NHS contract. To put it simply, doctors in Australia are paid more to work fewer hours.

For many who board planes to faraway hospitals, though, financial benefits and tax breaks are far from the forefront of their minds. Whether it's the beaches of Australia or South Africa, or the scenery of New Zealand, working as a doctor abroad provides the perfect excuse to gain an entirely new cultural experience and to travel the world.

Working as a junior doctor on a training scheme in the NHS can feel like a rat race, transferred between hospitals every few months with very little notice and living continually at the mercy of rota coordinators up and down the country. Pursuing options abroad can provide relief from this hamster-wheel existence, resetting priorities and reinvigorating any sagging enthusiasm.

WHERE CAN UK DOCTORS WORK?

In short, almost anywhere. Australia and New Zealand remain the most popular destinations for doctors moving abroad, but over the period of 2013–2016, certificates of good standing were issued for over 150 countries.

Just over 100 doctors applied for a certificate to cover the United States in 2016, possibly due to the more stringent entry requirements necessary to work in the US. In order to practice in the US, doctors must initially complete two stages of the United States Medical Licensing Examination (USMLE),[7] a challenging and not inexpensive process.

Australia has traditionally been the most popular destination for UK doctors seeking employment abroad, and for many years, gaps in their medical workforce were filled by overseas medics. Recently though, the tide has started to turn. New medical schools are opening in Australia, and every year more home grown doctors are being produced. There has been a concerted effort from the Australian government to curb the number of overseas doctors gaining employment in the country, limiting the numbers to 2100 annually,[8] and visa restrictions have also been tightened with removal of a number of occupations from the skilled occupation list.[9] There are still positions available, but the process has become considerably more difficult.

Beyond the administrative aspects to consider, there is one's professional development to bear in mind, too. As already discussed, there are other countries that share similar healthcare characteristics to the NHS, allowing the opportunity for career progression and a seamless return to practice in the UK, if required. Others, particularly those with more limited healthcare resources, require a vastly different approach to the art of medical practice. This can work in a doctor's favour, broadening their experience and providing a greater appreciation of the importance of resource management.

It can also make re-integration into a system such as the NHS more difficult, either due a prolonged absence from the familiarity of day-to-day practice, or through a changed attitude towards healthcare as a result of acclimatising to a new method of practice.

Language differences can of course preclude many UK doctors from working in a large proportion of countries, but generally if the will is there, it is possible to fashion a job opportunity in most hospitals in the world.

That is not to say that there isn't a significant amount of legwork required to orchestrate employment abroad. The process can be lengthy, complicated, and expensive. There are multiple factors to consider: medical registration, indemnity cover, and visa applications to name just a few. Each of these require supporting documentation, fees, and a large helping of patience. Fortunately, with so many doctors having trodden the same path before, there is a vast array of support and advice available (the BMA website and medicfootprints.org are good places to start).

EXTRA TRAINING

In many countries, no extra training is required. Obviously, if a job abroad requires a particular branch of medicine rarely encountered in the UK – tropical medicine for instance – then it can be useful to read up on potential clinical scenarios, but most medical skills are transferrable overseas without the need for further formal training.

The exception is the USMLE, as mentioned previously. This is a prerequisite for anyone hoping to work in the US. There are courses available to aid in preparation for this exam, available both in a classroom setting and online.

RETURNING TO NHS TRAINING

There are doctors everywhere that will warn against working abroad. There's a widely held belief that taking time out of training negatively impacts upon doctors' chances of progressing in their chosen career, the move supposedly demonstrating lack of commitment to their chosen specialty.

In truth, it's impossible to say for sure whether taking time away from training negatively impacts upon training opportunities. Certainly, experience in a relevant medical field and enhancement of clinical skills can be beneficial when it comes to demonstrating suitability for a training post, whereas a year spent sitting on a beach away from medicine may have the opposite effect.

There is no objective evidence that taking time out of the NHS to work abroad negatively impacts upon training prospects, and if planned and executed appropriately and with future career ambitions in mind, the process can be viewed by potential employers as a positive. Adaptability, experience, and the ability to work in new and challenging environments are attractive qualities in a prospective employee, and a rewarding experience working abroad can provide the opportunity to develop all of these skills.

The practicalities of returning to the training in the UK are also worth considering. NHS England has recently attempted to simplify the process for returning GPs, acknowledging that doctors in the past have been dissuaded from returning due to the bureaucracy associated with the exercise.[10] Those that spend two or more years out of training, though, will still require simulated surgeries and work-based assessments in order to work independently again in the UK.[11]

CASE STUDY

In the eight years since qualifying from medical school, I've worked abroad on two separate occasions, and for two vastly different reasons.

Finishing my foundation training in 2012, I still hadn't settled on a training programme that I was ready to pursue, and feeling as though I needed time away from training to make a decision, I drafted an email outlining my interest in working overseas and sent it out to hospitals all over the world. Barely two weeks later, and after the briefest of telephone interviews completed in the early hours of the morning, I had accepted an emergency medicine post in Melbourne, Australia.

Apart from the occasional spider bite, the day-to-day job and my own responsibilities were largely similar to the A&E job in FY2, only without the inhumane rota and terrible departmental morale. The makeup of the department was familiar too, staffed almost exclusively by British and Irish doctors. The Australian approach to emergency medicine – working up each patient more thoroughly before referring to specialities – offered a new challenge, and one which left me seriously considering A&E as an eventual career.

Meanwhile, away from the job, the experience was even more fulfilling. With more free time, I was able to enjoy everything that a new city and a new country offered. I embraced the outdoor culture of Australia fully, reacquainting myself with the active lifestyle that had fallen by the wayside throughout foundation training in the UK. I was surrounded by like-minded British medics, all with similar reasons for moving to the other side of the world, and with more disposable income, I was afforded the luxury of being able to travel, attend sporting events, and take the opportunity to make the most of everything Melbourne could offer.

Sadly, it wasn't to last. I'd only intended to move to Australia for a year, but six months earlier than expected, I was flying home. As much as I had been enjoying the experience, I fell ill a little over four months after arriving in the country. With no immediate prospect of returning to work and no family support in the same time zone, I was forced to make the difficult decision to give up on my plans for the year. I returned to the UK feeling like a failure, but with a pledge to myself that if I had the chance to work abroad again in the future, I'd grasp it with both hands.

Early in 2016, that very opportunity materialised. I was two years into GP training at this point and had to some degree given up on the idea of working abroad anytime in the near future. I had just finished another exhausting, unrelenting six months in A&E though, and was feeling as though I needed a change. It was only later on, and with the benefit of hindsight, that I realised that I was suffering from burnout.

Spurred on by a fellow trainee's experience during a year out of GP training, I submitted an application for an Out Of Programme Experience (OOPE), and to my surprise, was granted permission to take a year out between ST2 and ST3.

A few months later and I was packing my bags again, armed with my stethoscope and my Australian visa, this time bound for Sydney. I was to be working in A&E again, but this time as a registrar in charge of a busy emergency department overnight.

Despite the stress of increasing responsibility, within weeks I was settled back into the Australian way of life and was enjoying working as a doctor again. The job was challenging in terms of responsibility and decision making, but for the first time in a while, I felt valued as a member of the medical team, rather than merely a provider of a service. The night shifts in charge of the department and supervising less-experienced doctors were anxiety-inducing and exhausting, but once completed, left me with a sense of achievement and satisfaction. My new colleagues were supportive and inspiring, and at my six-monthly Skype review with my clinical supervisor in the UK, I was able to report a genuine feeling that I was progressing professionally and had regained an enthusiasm for a career in medicine.

I followed the crisis in the NHS and the ongoing junior doctors contract dispute from a distance with a mixture of sadness and guilt. If I am entirely honest though, seeing the pictures of patients queuing for hours in corridors and the solemn faces of my former colleagues I experienced another emotion: one of relief. The ingrained masochism I felt working in the NHS had been replaced by the sensation of job satisfaction and fulfilment.

A year away from training quickly became 18 months, and I seriously considered the option of dropping out of training in the UK altogether and making the move permanent. The Australian visa reforms worried me: If I left now, would this be my last chance to work in this country that I've grown to love?

In the end, though, I made the sensible decision: to return home and complete the final year of GP training. Whether this will become permanent or not, only time will tell. Australia will still be there, and hopefully with a postgraduate qualification under my belt, so will the job opportunities. If there is a next time, I might be saying goodbye to the NHS for good.

CONCLUSION

Choosing to work abroad can be emotionally satisfying and professionally rewarding. Whether time out away from the UK is just to provide some breathing space to think about long-term career options or is a more permanent move, it is unlikely to be something you regret. There are inevitable bureaucratic obstacles to be overcome but the rewards beyond the obstacles will more than compensate and may leave you reinvigorated and enjoying medicine again.

REFERENCES

1. UK Foundation Programme Career Destination Report 2017. Available: www.foundationprogramme.nhs.uk. Accessed: 19th August 2018.
2. Rimmer, A. 2017. Half of doctors don't go straight into specialty training. *BMJ* 356: j672.

3. Chowdhury, M. 2016. Freedom of Information request to the GMC. Available: https://www.whatdotheyknow.com/request/number_of_certificates_of_good_s. Accessed: 19th August 2018.

4. Merrick R. 2016. Jeremy Hunt Unveils Plans to Fine Junior Doctors Who Move Abroad After Training The independent 4th October 2016. Available: https://www.independent.co.uk/news/uk/politics/jeremy-hunt-plans-to-fine-doctors-who-move-abroad-after-training-a7343531.html. Accessed 15th September 2018.

5. Smith SE et al. 2018. Foundation Year 2 doctors' reasons for leaving UK medicine: An in-depth analysis of decision-making using semistructured interviews. *BMJ Open* 8: e019456.

6. Doward J. 2015. New Doctors Leave the NHS for Better Life Abroad. The Guardian 23rd August 2015. Available: https://www.theguardian.com/society/2015/aug/23/new-doctors-leave-nhs-for-better-life-abroad. Accessed 15th September 2018.

7. Education Commission for Foreign Medical Graduates. Website: www.ecfmg.org. Accessed 15th September 2018.

8. The Guardian. 2018. Australia to Let in Fewer Overseas Doctors. The Guardian 8th May 2018. Available: https://www.theguardian.com/australia-news/2018/may/08/australia-federal-budget-2018-doctors-overseas-health-medical-training-regions. Accessed 15th September 2018.

9. Financial Times. Australia curbs flow of disgruntled UK junior doctors. Available: https://www.ft.com/content/38513e9a-a029-11e6-86d5-4e36b35c3550. Accessed 15th September 2018.

10. National GP induction and refresher scheme. NHS England. https://www.england.nhs.uk/gp/gpfv/workforce/returning-to-practice/gp-induction/. Accessed 15th September 2018.

11. NHS Website. Thinking of Returning to General Practice? Available: http://www.gpreturner.nhs.uk/. Accessed 15th September 2018.

8

Resilience

EUAN LAWSON

What is resilience? How do know if you've got it? And if you haven't got it then how do you develop it?

There are few easy answers to these questions, but there is an emerging consensus on some of the factors.

When the term resilience is applied to materials, it refers to a quality that allows for it to be bent, stretched, or compressed and still return to its original shape. Amongst doctors, it has been defined as 'the individual's ability to adapt to and manage stress and adversity'.[1]

Southwick and Charney have studied the quality of resilience in people who have been through trauma, both physical and psychological, in contexts as diverse as fighting in a warzone or being the victim of sexual assault. They noted that resilience is 'complex, multidimensional and dynamic in nature'.[2]

Resilience is not a fixed commodity. It can vary across the life course, it can vary from month to month even, and it can also vary depending on the exact nature of the stressor.

NEUROBIOLOGY OF RESILIENCE

This is worth dwelling on. One might assume resilience is a rather nebulous, new-age term related to aspects of personality or other inner qualities that are difficult to define. However, neuroscientists are increasingly able to map out the specific neural pathways involved in resilience, and this leads to credible strategies to address concerns when those pathways bend or break.

The acute stress response

This is how the mind and body respond to persistent stress. We all know the hormones that rise in these circumstances. The fight-or-flight surge of adrenaline and catecholamines. The rise in cortisol levels and also in pro-inflammatory cytokines. These are primitive responses, enormously helpful in the course of evolution to preserve us from short-term hazards. When the stresses are persistent, as so often in modern life, these responses do not necessarily ebb away, and this prolonged stress activation can cause significant damage with changes in the brain tissue and maladaptation in the hypothalamic–pituitary–adrenal axis. This can then lead to chronic illnesses, including cardiovascular disease.

The problem with sustained stress is that it impairs decision making. Martin et al. highlight other impacts:[3]

- Interference with empathy and communication
- Narrowing of the field of vision (literally and metaphorically)
- Decrease in generosity
- Decrease in cooperativeness
- Increase in xenophobia
- Increased likelihood of interpreting ambiguous expressions as hostile
- Increased likelihood of displacing frustration and aggression onto those around us

In other words, 'it makes us more dull-witted and less friendly'.[4] Compassion and empathy diminish, and this, clearly, is not ideal for anybody working in the medical profession.

PHYSICIAN PERSONALITY AND RESILIENCE

Physician personality has been found to be associated with wellness. One Norwegian study found that neuroticism and conscientiousness traits predict stress in medical students.[5] Workaholism and perfectionism have been associated with suicide in physicians.[6] In a cross-sectional study of over 1000 Canadian physicians, Lemaire and Wallace explored how personality types related to doctors' perceptions of wellbeing and occupational performance.[7] They noted that physicians tended to identify strongly with three different personality types: workaholic, 'type A personality' (competitive and ambitious), and 'control freak' personality.

The workaholic personality was associated with one potentially harmful and three positive wellbeing outcomes. The control freak personality was associated with five potentially harmful outcomes. Personality type is key to determining overall resilience.

There is also a culture within medicine that can exacerbate existing personality traits in doctors and medical students. Personalities themselves may not be malleable, but awareness amongst students and doctors of their own potential vulnerabilities and their inherent resilience and ability to withstand burnout is crucial to managing clinician wellness. You may not be able to stop being a control freak, but an awareness that this can put you at higher risk of burnout will help you mitigate this risk.

OTHER FEATURES ASSOCIATED WITH RESILIENCE

Charney and Southwick found 10 factors associated with resilience.[2] Psychological and social factors associated with resilience include

- Facing fear: An adaptive response
- Having a moral compass

- Religion and spirituality
- Social support
- Having good role models
- Being physically fit
- Brain fitness: Making sure your brain is challenged
- Having 'cognitive and emotional flexibility'
- Having 'meaning, purpose, and growth' in life
- 'Realistic' optimism

This is perhaps more encouraging than the previous study relating to personality traits because these are not all necessarily fixed traits. They can, potentially, be addressed.

'Realistic' optimism

What do we mean by optimism? Southwick and Charney regard this as a 'future orientated attitude'. Optimists tend to believe that the future will be bright and that good things will happen to people who work hard.

Psychologists have developed tests to measure optimism. Some of the most resilient people that have been studied have been the most optimistic. Psychologists have investigated why optimists seem to be particularly resilient. These studies lead us back to the fight-or-flight reaction described above, because it has been shown that when we experience positive emotions our level of physiological arousal is reduced. This is a direct biological mechanism to ensure that people benefit from their optimism. This in turn results in improved attention and an improved ability to actively problem solve, as well as a greater interest in socialising. These are useful benefits for those working in medicine.

Facing fear: An adaptive response

This is another factor associated with resilience that is linked to the fight-or-flight response. Pavlov's dogs and the phenomenon of classical conditioning are familiar to most people and, just like Pavlov's dogs, we may experience a response such as fear when exposed to a stimulus which would not otherwise cause distress but has been previously associated with some kind of traumatic event. This resilience-associated factor is particularly important to people who have had a very traumatic experience in the past and may therefore be conditioned to experience a strong emotional response to similar stimuli in the future.

Ethics and altruism: Having a moral compass

When Southwick and Charney interviewed people who had been through trauma they found that many of the individuals who seem to be particularly resilient had a sense of right and wrong that was particularly valuable to them during periods of extreme stress. They also found that altruism, the concern for the welfare of others, was often part of that value system. Some trauma survivors, particularly those who had been involved in torture, had been forced to face some deeply difficult moral choices and having a moral compass to guide these choices was beneficial. Arguably, a moral compass is embedded within the medical profession where there is a strong code of moral and ethical behaviour; however, there is value in medical students and doctors consciously engaging with that moral compass when confronted with difficult decisions.

Religion and spirituality

Many people find that their religious beliefs offer them resilience. Southwick and Charney felt this to be as applicable to people who are atheists as to those with strongly held beliefs in any of the world's major religions. Importantly, this factor is not concerned with a belief in a particular god, rather it is about people feeling comfortable with their place in the universe as a result of their belief system.

Social support

Man is basically a social creature. Having a social support network has been shown to be positively associated with resilience.

Social support can promote physical and mental health, and the relationship seems to work both ways – it may in fact be the case that giving social support is even more beneficial for physical health than receiving it. There is a particular biology of relationships, and neuroscientists have been able to demonstrate specific neurobiological changes that occur in the context of relationships. For example, the hormone oxytocin seems to play a strong role in social communication and the formation of a sense of affiliation, as well as in other interactions such as sexual behaviour.

On the face of it, medicine seems like a highly social activity but, as discussed in earlier chapters, it is entirely possible for doctors to become very isolated, particularly when working erratic shift patterns. The interactions we have with patients are not necessarily social, and it is possible for junior doctors to go for prolonged periods in a busy job without any social interaction meaningful enough to promote their own good health.

Wallace and Lemaire studied positive and negative factors associated with physician wellbeing and noted the importance of co-worker support. Interestingly, this study also highlighted the role of patients in wellbeing. While being a source of stress, they were also an important source of satisfaction, and therefore wellbeing, for doctors.[8]

Having good role models

In some of the first studies to look at resilience, it was shown that the most resilient children usually had at least one person who gave them genuine support and served as a role model. Southwick and Charney have found similar findings in their own research. Their research has shown that everybody needs appropriate, resilient role models. Mentors form the critical role in inspiring and motivating their charges and fostering resilience. How does it work? This seems to be down to imitation – an innate ability and one that we have from the earliest infancy but that persists throughout our lives. Role modelling has been well established in medical education and for trainees at all levels, but, perhaps, there could be further development of this area for more senior clinicians.

Being physically fit

The obvious benefits of physical exercise to our physical health seem also to extend to benefits to mental health, including improvements to mood and cognition. Most importantly, for our purposes, there seems to be benefit in terms of resilience. There are clear neurobiological mechanisms that explain how this could function. The chemicals that improve mood such as endorphins, serotonin, and dopamine are all increased after exercise. In addition, the pathways that release cortisol are dampened by exercise. There are other potential mechanisms including neurogenesis (making of new brain cells when specific genes are switched on).

One of the key points to remember about exercise and resilience is that we only get stronger and more physically fit by ensuring we have appropriate rest periods. This is often neglected. Physical exercise itself is the stressor but the adaptation only comes afterwards. This means diet and sleep are key factors in developing resilience due to physical activity.

Brain fitness: Making sure your brain is challenged

Southwick and Charney found that people who are lifelong learners tend to have higher levels of resilience. They found that certain activities can promote both cognitive and emotional improvements in brain function – mental training. There is still some scepticism around 'brain training', but there is good evidence that there is an enormous amount of inherent plasticity in the brain, and this neuroplasticity can be developed in some form. It is also known that the use of techniques such as mindfulness can help us learn how to develop calm and an improved awareness of our emotions and perceptions. Even if people remain sceptical about interventions such as mindfulness, there is clear evidence for cognitive behavioural therapy, an obvious form of mental and emotional training.

Having cognitive and emotional flexibility

Cognitive flexibility is an important factor in resilience. We need to have the ability to accept the reality of the situations that we are in. It is obvious that avoidance and denial are not helpful in coping with changing circumstances. This concept of 'acceptance' has been identified by psychologists as an important ingredient in people being able to tolerate highly stressful circumstances. It has also been shown to be associated with better psychological and physical health.

This is been described by Southwick and Charney as cognitive reappraisal. Cognitive reappraisal can come in a number of different forms. One potential area is in the shape of gratitude. Resilient people that have been through particularly traumatic events often then appreciate the things they still have. It is also suggested that humour is a form of cognitive reappraisal as it is a mechanism to help people reframe events and to face their fears and thus using humour can be a way to boost our resilience.

Having 'meaning, purpose, and growth' in life

The tenth factor described by Southwick and Charney is about having a purpose. Those people who have a clear sense of mission often have a very deep resilience and ability to withstand enormous stresses and strains. In many ways, in the UK, the NHS has provided many clinicians with that sense of purpose in their clinical practice. It gives many workers in the NHS a meaning that goes beyond the monthly pay packet. This factor also highlights a potential unintended consequence of reorganisations and stress within the NHS system; it will, indirectly, erode the resilience of the workers within it. Conversely, working within teams and departments for whom we feel loyalty will enhance this sense of purpose.

THE PARADOX

One of the biggest challenges facing the medical profession is the fundamental paradox at the heart of managing burnout. There is an expectation that doctors will be cool, calm, and collected, confident and yet still caring and empathetic.

These may not be obviously mutually exclusive, but the neurobiology of the human brain rather suggests that, to some extent, they are exactly that. Doctors are faced with people going through tremendously intense emotional experiences while unwell. Yet clinicians need to suppress the parts of the brain – limbic and reptilian – that regard these experiences as highlighting a threat. Patients push our limbic brain buttons, even if it is happening subconsciously.

Resilience is our ability to soak up that neurobiological stress and not develop the adverse consequences of persistent stress and arousal. The need to develop resilience in trainees has been recognised. In one study, GP trainees on a scheme in the south of England were found to have significant levels of burnout in their first year of training.[9]

If the innate resilience of doctors is being stretched at this early stage in their careers, it suggests that we need to start building on that innate resilience at medical school, during training, and on through our careers, in order to future proof ourselves against the increasing stresses of our working lives.

REFERENCES

1. Lown M, Lewith G, Simon C, Peters D. 2015. Resilience: What is it, why do we need it, and can it help us? *Br J Gen Pract.* 65(639): e708–e710.
2. Southwick SM, Charney DS. 2012. *Resilience: The Science of Mastering Life's Greatest Challenges. Resilience: The Science of Mastering Life's Greatest Challenges.* New York: Cambridge University Press.
3. Martin LJ et al. 2015. Reducing social stress elicits emotional contagion of pain in mouse and human strangers. *Curr Biol.* 25(3): 326–332.
4. Peters D. 2016. *The Neurobiology of Resilience.* InnovAiT. SAGE Publications Sage UK: London; 9(6): 333–341.
5. Tyssen R, Dolatowski FC, Røvik JO, Thorkildsen RF, Ekeberg HE, Gude T, Grønvold NT, Vaglum P. 2007. Personality traits and types predict medical school stress: A six-year longitudinal and nationwide study. *Medical Education.* 41(8): 781–787.

6. Beevers CG, Miller IW. 2004. Perfectionism, cognitive bias, and hopelessness as prospective predictors of suicidal ideation. *Suicide and Life-Threat Behav.* 34(2): 126–137.

7. Lemaire JB, Wallace JE. 2014. How physicians identify with predetermined personalities and links to perceived performance and wellness outcomes: A cross-sectional study. *BMC Health Serv Res.* 14: 616.

8. Wallace JE, Lemaire J. 2007. On physician well being-you'll get by with a little help from your friends. *Soc Sci Med.* 64(12): 2565–2577.

9. Sales B, Macdonald A, Scallan S, Crane S. 2016. How can educators support general practice (GP) trainees to develop resilience to prevent burnout? *Educ Prim Care.* 27(6): 487–493.

9

Finding help

FIONA DAY

This chapter covers interventions for junior doctors who want to take proactive action to build their resilience, as well as sources of help for those who are concerned about their own wellbeing and are in need of professional help. The evidence base for what works to prevent and recover from burnout is growing all the time, and the good news is that there are lots of things you can do to help yourself if you are starting to feel the pressure.

THERAPEUTIC HELP

Medical

All doctors in the UK should be registered with a general practitioner (GP) who will normally be the first point of contact for any significant health-related concerns. It's well documented that doctors find it difficult to seek help from another doctor and that some doctors find it difficult to treat doctors as patients rather than as colleagues, and these are well recognised barriers to doctors getting the help they need. However, if you are concerned about your own wellbeing, then your GP would normally be your first point of contact for a confidential assessment and discussion about your health.

It is vitally important that you don't self-diagnose or attempt to self-treat if you or someone else is concerned that you may have more than a passing, mild mental-health concern. It's also really important to be honest with your GP; doctors often end up denying themselves the help that they need because they know how to say 'the right things' to make things appear better than they are. As with most conditions, the earlier you seek and gain the treatment you need, the quicker your recovery is likely to be. It can be difficult for many doctors to seek help as it may bring about feelings of shame, vulnerability, and failure, and seeking help is always the right thing to do.

Your GP will coordinate any other services that you need, if required. If you are a GP or GP trainee in England, you may be able to access the NHS-funded private health service called the GP Health Service, or alternatively your employer may be willing to pay for you to use the Practitioner Health Programme. Both of these are run by a private medical group, the Hurley Group.

Psychological

We are very fortunate that there is now a wide range of highly effective, evidence-based psychological interventions in the form of cognitive behaviour therapy (CBT) which are available through local 'IAPT' (Increasing Access to Psychological Therapies) services. These can be accessed directly or via primary care. There are also a large number of CBT therapists who work privately across the UK in person and online.

There is no statutory regulation of psychotherapists and counsellors, some of whom may be CBT trained, though there is regulation of practising psychologists, who may also be CBT trained. You should check that they are accredited as a CBT therapist (with the British Association for Behavioural and Cognitive Psychotherapies, for example).

There is growing evidence that 'third wave', mindfulness-based approaches to CBT such as acceptance and commitment therapy (ACT) can produce longer-lasting improvements;[1] you may want to discuss with your CBT therapist which models they use in their clinical practice.

Substance misuse and other addictions

Many doctors turn to alcohol, recreational and prescribed drugs to cope with difficult feelings such as those of burnout. Many doctors also become involved in other addictive behaviours such as gambling. If you are worried about whether you have an addiction, you can seek help through your GP, or your local IAPT service will be able to direct you to specialist addiction services in your local area. Professional help with this will be vital to your recovery.

NON-THERAPEUTIC PROFESSIONAL HELP

Coaching and mentoring

Coaching and mentoring are both very valuable personal and professional development opportunities which are widely available within the NHS and on a private basis. They have several aspects in common and also differ in several ways from each other. Both rely on a 1:1 relationship based on trust and conducted through a series of conversations which aim to develop the personal or professional competencies of the client.

According to the European Coaching and Mentoring Council,[2] coaching and mentoring are defined as:

A professionally guided process that inspires clients to maximise their personal and professional potential. It is a structured, purposeful and transformational process, helping clients to see and test alternative ways for improvement of competence, decision making and enhancement of quality of life. Coach and Mentor and client work together in a partnering relationship on strictly confidential terms. In this relationship, clients are experts on the content & decision making level; the coach & mentor is an expert in professionally guiding the process.

A professional accredited Coach is an expert in establishing a relationship with people in a series of conversations with the purpose of: Serving the clients to improve their performance or enhance their personal development or both, choosing their own goals and ways of doing it; Interacting with each person or group by applying one or more relevant methods, according to standards and ethical principles set up by EMCC and other professional associations.

Mentoring is a developmental process, which may in some forms involve a transfer of skill or knowledge from a more experienced person to a less experienced, through learning, dialogue and role modelling. In other forms may be a partnership for mutual learning between peers or across differences such as age, race or discipline.

An experienced coach will work with you to make changes to your working life and career to help you to get more meaning, purpose, satisfaction, and an improved sense of wellbeing. A typical coaching intervention would be four, 90-minute coaching sessions over a 3–4 month period, with you working between sessions to understand yourself, experiment with different behaviours, make requests of other people, and learn new skills to improve your wellbeing and resilience. Many coaches are skilled at helping people to cope with their current jobs, return to work after a period of sickness absence, and/or change career direction within or outside of medicine.

If you want to consider career coaching, be aware that coaching is still an unregulated area of professional practice. You are advised to check that the coach is fully qualified: minimum ILM5 coaching certificate, member of a coaching professional body, has professional and public liability insurance, is a registered Data Controller, is in supervision one hour per 20 hours of coaching with a qualified supervisor, undertakes continuing professional development (CPD), and that you feel they are competent and experienced to help you with your specific situation. Professional coaching takes place within a contract, an agreement between the coach and the client which creates a safe place for a deep level of personal and professional learning to occur. Some coaches work within the NHS; however many people seek an external coach due to their impartiality and objectivity.

There is a lot of informal mentoring within the NHS from senior colleagues. This can be a great help to many doctors, but if there is no contract or agreement between the two parties, then things can sometimes get a bit messy in terms of conflicts of interest. That is why many people will use an external coach who they can feel confident that they can tell the good, the bad, and the ugly to in terms of their own experiences, and their experiences within the organisation. Mentors generally have a 'sponsorship' role within your career, and it may not always be appropriate to tell them the whole story as you experience it.

SELF-HELP

This section is not a substitute for clinical assessment and care but is designed to help you to take action to improve your own wellbeing.

Understanding your mind

For all that we are highly trained doctors, most of us don't understand our own minds from a more psychological perspective. Here is a simple model to help you.

Every human being on this planet has a brain which has evolved over millennia to be hardwired to constantly scan for danger, to keep us 'in the tribe' rather than on our own in the wilderness, and to seek rewards necessary for our survival and the survival of our genes. Thanks to different stages of evolution, we have three basic emotional regulation systems.[3] The oldest one is a threat-focused system, helping us to constantly scan for danger. Then there is a drive state pushing us to seek rewards. The third one is a system which helps us to build relationships with others and to relax and unwind, often called an affiliative, or soothing, system.

From an evolutionary perspective, our human brains are well-adapted to the environment in which humans have lived through most of history and were probably great in stone-age survival conditions. However, in the chronic, low-level stressful environment of the twenty-first century, our brains often don't work so well, especially if we have inherited genes which put us at greater risk of developing mental-health problems, or if we've had traumatic early-life or adult-life experiences. In essence, modern life, and perhaps particularly modern life in the medical profession, puts every one of us at risk of burnout and related mental-health conditions.

The good news is that cognitive neuropsychology is teaching us that we can consciously use our minds to change our brains for the better – and that is no small revolution in terms of understanding how you can use this evolving science to help you to prevent or recover from burnout.

Here is a set of interrelated brain training skills, which use the principles of positive neuroplasticity to help you. They are not mutually exclusive but will work in synergy to help you to get up the 'upward spiral'. The evidence base for this type of brain training is underdeveloped at the moment when compared with the level of evidence that you might expect for a clinical intervention, but they are all included because there is sufficient practice-based evidence or sufficient evidence in populations other than doctors to justify their inclusion, and the risk of harm is low and the potential for benefit is high.

1. Mindfulness training

Mindfulness is everywhere and yet virtually nowhere at the moment. It is one of the most misused words on the planet! There is a lot of hype about it being a panacea for all ills and also that to do it properly you need to have lots of props, to go on long retreats, and to learn to chant. In this section, I'll dispel some of the myths but also show you why psychologists and mental-health specialists are so excited about mindfulness.

I will be drawing on the evidence base, but not presenting a review of the evidence, in part because research in this field is still in its infancy. If mindfulness were a drug, you can be sure that there would be plenty of high-quality, internationally renowned papers in the field; however, because it isn't, there has not been a huge amount of funding into mindfulness based interventions (MBIs). Despite this, there are early suggestions that certain types of focused attention, awareness, and concentration practices ('mindfulness') can be effective as a transdiagnostic mental-health, substance-misuse, and behaviour-change intervention. I predict that in 50 years' time we will be able to tailor specific interventions for specific behavioural and mental-health conditions but, at the moment, 'mindfulness' is a pretty blunt tool. If you want to read a really good review of the evidence in an accessible format then buy yourself Goleman and Davidson's book *Altered Traits*[4] – you won't be disappointed.

Mindfulness is a method of training conscious awareness and attention. There are many different ways of doing this, all with different outcomes. One of the key skills to be learned is 'metacognitive introspective awareness', the ability to know what 'the mind' (attention and peripheral awareness) is focusing on at any moment in time. Through knowing what the mind is focusing on, we can learn to make wise choices about how to respond next, a skill which is key, for example, to managing ruminative thoughts of depression and thus preventing depression relapse.

Knowing what our minds are focusing on is not always a comfortable experience, and for many of us, we would rather not be aware of what was previously a more unconscious process. However, by being aware of our mental processes on a more regular basis, we can learn to notice the state of our minds in relation to the drive/anxiety states, and from this noticing of the habits of our mind, we can increasingly learn to make choices both in the moment and in the longer term, which bring us closer to the things which really matter in our lives.

Some schools teach that the sole purpose of mindfulness is to develop metacognitive introspective awareness. Other schools also believe that relaxation, equanimity, and 'awakening' are important aspects of mindfulness training. Personally, I think that if you don't enjoy the practice, you won't commit to it and progress, so I think it is important to enjoy and savour any feelings of relaxation, but not to allow this to become an opportunity to sleep or just to switch off. If you're tired, sleep, and when you're less tired, practice learning mindfulness, or use ways to learn mindfulness other than sitting or lying with your eyes closed, such as walking or listening to sounds.

Some schools emphasise learning to 'still the mind' over time and effort (it took me about 25 years before I could do this with any consistency!); others do not believe that stilling the mind is possible or desirable for most people. I believe that this is a skill that everyone can learn over time, but it takes diligence and patience and stilling the mind isn't the only benefit which mindfulness training can offer. For some people, mindfulness training is the first step in a journey of personal development.

Mindfulness can be practiced informally using everyday activities as a way to learn the skill of attention training and understanding the habits of your mind. Examples would be: listening to a piece of music; walking slowly in the park and paying attention to the experiences of the five senses or noticing where your mind wanders to; paying attention in a conversation through mindful listening; fully engaging in a domestic chore or a task at hand such as showering, preparing food, eating, or playing with children.

Practicing mindfulness formally means consciously choosing to temporarily suspend other activities in order to learn the skill of mindfulness through meditation. This may be sitting, walking, lying, or standing, but is usually practiced sitting in an upright chair or lying on a mat on the floor (rather than a bed, which is too inviting to fall asleep). There are lots of guided recorded practices which you may like to use to help you; however, here is a very basic practice you might like to try:

- Commit to finding 10 minutes on your own and undisturbed, ask others to not disturb you, switch off your mobile phone etc.
- Sit in an upright chair with your feet flat on the floor, hip width apart, head pointing up to the ceiling, in a relaxed but

not casual position, take a moment to get comfortable and symmetrical.

- Keep your eyes open or slowly lower your eyelids until they are closed.
- Take a moment to enjoy the feeling of slowing down and taking time for yourself.
- Become aware of the sounds around you, notice them without judging them, observe how they come and go.
- Bring your attention to the feeling of your body sitting in the chair, the points of contact of your body and the chair.
- When you notice your mind wandering, it's just the mind doing its job, bring your attention back to the feeling of contact between your body and the chair, the whole body sitting here right now.
- When you're ready, open your eyes, and reflect on the experience you had today.

You may like to buy the book *Mindfulness: A Practical Guide to Finding Peace in a Frantic World* by Mark Williams and Danny Penman.[5] The book has a free CD which is also available online for free from their website or as a free app. The best way to get a good grounding in the basics of mindfulness is to attend an eight-week course; this may be difficult as a junior doctor or medical student, but is something to work towards when you are in a position to do this. Ensure the teacher is fully qualified through the UK Mindfulness Network and note that most eight-week courses require 40–60 minutes of home practice most days of the week if you want to really learn these skills.

2. Developing self-compassion

Building compassion for oneself is a key skill which can also be extended to developing compassion for other people. By learning to be more kind to ourselves, we can still succeed in our careers and lives, but in a more sustainable way. It's like being your own best friend: when things are difficult, instead of blaming ourselves constantly, we can apologise and learn from our mistakes without adding to it by then spending hours or years berating ourselves for our inadequacies.

We all have the same basic brain, hardwired for survival in the Stone Age. We all make mistakes and get things wrong. As doctors, we are expected to get things right every time, and this is a really difficult mindset to live with. Self-compassion is a perfect counter to medical perfectionism, and knowing what 'good enough' is in any situation is vital for our long-term psychological health. Good enough for a GP may be 'safety netting' (come back in a few weeks if you're not better), 'good enough' in an emergency or acute system may be harder to assess.

Getting really clear feedback from your senior colleagues is vital to knowing what good enough is in any clinical situation. Ask for specific feedback to help you to know where the line is. You may aspire to excellence in every clinical encounter, but it should always be good enough (and it may well be excellent). Knowing what's enough and delivering this is your goal, not being perfect every waking moment. There are some great exercises to help you to develop self-compassion. See *The Compassionate Mind Foundation* website for their great resources and audio practices including 'soothing rhythm breathing' and other compassion focused exercises.[6]

3. *Team 'you'*

We all need a team of people around us to support and champion us through the ups and downs of life. Who is in your own team, and how can you build connections with people in the team and build the team over time? It's easy to get into a 'bunker mentality' of being independent and coping on your own. Get into the habit of turning towards people when things are difficult and sharing in others' joy and pain. Feeling loved and loving helps to activate your soothing system and builds stronger relationships for the future.

4. *Lifestyle and sleep*

Physical activity is a great boost for mental health and wellbeing, especially when it is outside in the fresh air or nature. How can you get more exercise into your life? Start with where you are at now, and try to identify something small and manageable that you can commit to. Getting enough high-quality sleep is a challenge for every doctor, and if you are having trouble sleeping, then you may like Guy Meadow's *The Sleep Book*.[7] Making sure you eat properly and using recreational substances like alcohol in moderation only are good habits to get into for life.

Management support

Your employer has duties under the Health at Work Act (1972) and other statutory health, safety, and welfare legislation and regulations. The employer is required to take reasonably practical action to do this, including assessing risks to their employees and acting on the risk assessment. If you are at risk of psychological harm through your work, the employer would be expected to show what reasonable action it has taken to protect you, the larger the organisation, the more effort is expected by the courts.

If you feel that you are at increased risk of psychological harm for whatever reason, you may wish to discuss this with your manager or human resources officer and ask for a personalised risk assessment. There are tools available to support managers in this process on the Health and Safety Executive website, or there may be internal processes which your line manager will need to follow. If your line manager doesn't know that you are struggling or at increased risk, or that you may have a disability (see below), then they can't help you as much as you may need. It's always best to seek support at an early stage before you get more seriously ill. A risk assessment for 'stress at work' would normally cover six areas:[8]

1. *Demands*: This includes issues such as workload, work patterns, and the work environment.
2. *Control*: How much say the person has in the way they do their work.
3. *Support*: This includes the encouragement, sponsorship, and resources provided by the organisation, line management, and colleagues.
4. *Relationships*: This includes promoting positive working to avoid conflict and dealing with unacceptable behaviour.

5. *Role*: Whether or not people understand their role within the organisation and whether or not the organisation ensures that they do not have conflicting roles.
6. *Change*: How organisational change (large or small) is managed and communicated in the organisation.

OCCUPATIONAL HEALTH AND THE EQUALITY ACT 2010

There is a lot of misinformation about occupational health. Occupational health services for NHS staff operate separately from NHS services, the records are kept in a separate confidential system, and information can only be shared with your employer or another person, including your GP, with your consent unless there is grave concern about your health or the impact of your health on your work, or concern that another person is at risk, or when requested by law. Even then, you will normally have been encouraged to self-report before any member of the occupational health team breaks your confidence. There are extensive guidelines for occupational health clinicians relating to protecting your confidentiality.

BOX 9.1: Other sources of help

There are other places you may be able to get help and these include

- The General Medical Council
- The BMA
- The National Clinical Assessment Service. Website: www.ncas.nhs.uk
- ACAS (Advisory, Conciliation and Arbitration Service). Website: www.acas.org.uk/index.aspx?articleid=1461
- Doctors Support Network. Website: www.dsn.org.uk/support-for-doctors
- MIND. Website: www.mind.org.uk
- Samaritans. Website: www.samaritans.org

Some occupational health departments have access to therapeutic interventions, perhaps tailored to the needs of healthcare professionals, or perhaps available in a more timely fashion than standard NHS services. This is not always the case and some occupational health providers within the NHS focus more on assessments and advice for employers. Being honest about the severity of the problem will enable the occupational health team to give your employer the most appropriate advice to keep you in work and to keep you healthy. It is worth remembering that if the NHS did not employ healthcare staff with a history of burnout or mild, moderate, and/or severe mental illness, there would not be many people left to work within the NHS! It is important that you don't see yourself as a failure or unemployable; all cases are assessed on a person-by-person basis, and most people can be successfully supported or rehabilitated back into the workplace.

The Equality Act 2010[9] was introduced as a key piece of legislation to protect people with a variety of 'protected characteristics', of which one is disability. An occupational health clinician will advise your employer as to whether they believe that the Equality Act is likely to apply in your specific case. Occupational health can only advise the employer about whether they believe the Equality Act is likely to apply, the only way that the Equality Act can be properly tested in reality is by an Employment Tribunal (a special court where an employee can ask for a ruling on whether they have been unfairly discriminated against because of a disability). An Employment Tribunal will use four 'tests' to determine whether you are likely to have a disability which is protected by the Equality Act.

You are considered to have a disability under the Equality Act 2010 if you have:

1. A physical or mental impairment
2. That has a 'substantial' and
3. 'Long-term' negative effect
4. On your ability to do normal daily activities

The Equality Act 2010 protects you if you have a disability and covers areas including:

- Application forms
- Interview arrangements

- Aptitude or proficiency tests
- Job offers
- Terms of employment, including pay
- Promotion, transfer, and training opportunities
- Dismissal or redundancy
- Discipline and grievances

If you are likely to be considered disabled under the Equality Act 2010, your employer is required to make reasonable adjustments to support you in the workplace. The bigger the employer, the more extensive the Employment Tribunal would expect the reasonable adjustments to be. The NHS is obviously a large employer and would be expected to show that they had made reasonable adjustments to support you if you are likely to be considered disabled.

CONCLUSION

Understanding yourself and your own mind is crucial if you are to prevent and to recover from burnout. There are many evidence-based interventions to help you, so get into action today and start the journey to better mental health and wellbeing for the rest of your life.

REFERENCES

1. Zettle RD, Hayes SC, Barnes-Holmes D, Biglan A. 2015. *The Wiley Handbook of Contextual Behaviour Science.* New Jersey: Wiley.
2. Website: https://emccuk.org/Public/Resources/ Competence_Framework/Public/1Resources/ Competence_Framework.aspx?hkey=ad98bd86-8bb8- 4435-913d-5258f6774375. Accessed 2nd May 2018.
3. Gilbert P. 2009. *The Compassionate Mind.* London: Constable & Robinson.
4. Goleman D, Davidson RJ. 2017. *Altered Traits: Science Reveals How Meditation Changes Your Mind, Brain, and Body.* New York: Avery.

5. Williams M, Penman D. 2011. *Mindfulness: A Practical Guide to Finding Peace in a Frantic World*. London: Piatkus.
6. The Compassionate Mind Foundation. Website: compassionatemind.co.uk/resources Accessed: 19th August 2018.
7. Meadows G. 2014. *The Sleep Book*. London: Orion Publishing Co.
8. Health and Safety Executive. What are the Management Standards? Available: www.hse.gov.uk/stress/standards/index.htm. Accessed: 19th August 2018.
9. The Equality Act. 2010. Available: www.gov.uk/definition-of-disability-under-equality-act-2010. Accessed: 19th August 2018.

10

Final thoughts

ADAM STATEN

The issue of sick and suffering medical students and doctors is an uncomfortable one. We are supposed to be the cool head of compassion, able to help those in need without ever needing help ourselves. This has been the aspiration, even the expectation, of the medical profession for centuries, and yet the evidence suggests that our own neurobiology makes this all but unattainable. If we are truly to show compassion and feel empathy for our patients, it is simply not possible to remain completely psychologically unaffected by the suffering of our patients. We cannot expect to spend our working lives sharing in the physical, psychological, and emotional pain of our patients and yet retain our air of detached concern.

Some degree of burnout should be seen as inevitable, or at least highly probable, unless we take active measures to prevent it or remedy it. The statistics back this up with physicians having been shown to suffer from burnout across healthcare systems, across specialisms, and through the age range of those practising and studying medicine. In 2012, a survey of American physicians found that 60% would retire immediately if they were able.[1]

In 2017, the Royal College of Anaesthetists surveyed 2300 trainees and found 85% of them to be at risk of burnout.[2] The Practitioner Health Programme – a service for doctors suffering with mental health and addiction problems – has treated over 3000 doctors in a decade, with representatives amongst their patients from all specialties.[3] This growing body of evidence is hard to ignore. The evidence that signs of burnout develop at medical school, before a budding doctor has ever treated a patient, is perhaps even more worrying.

These figures show how widespread the problem is, and tell us that we must not see burnout as a problem experienced by individuals but as the product of the job we do and the systems within which we work. Whilst the effects of burnout may be a personal tragedy, when the syndrome is so common, it is ultimately the system, and the patients that it serves, that suffer because of it. The problem is systemic.

The solution, then, must also be systemic.

Recognising that many of us have psychological traits that predispose us to burnout, learning how to spot the symptoms at an early stage, and knowing how to build our mental resilience and how to treat ourselves when we our suffering are all useful, but ultimately, they are just reactive responses to an entirely predictable problem.

An awareness of burnout, and an awareness of the means by which we can stave it off, should be built into the way we learn, the way we train, and the way we work. Many medical schools, primarily in the US, are already recognising this and building resilience modules into their curricula, and the tools available to make our lives at work more tolerable – Balint groups, Schwartz Rounds, mentorship programmes for example – already exist but are not yet widely practiced.

The changes described above are not seismic in themselves, but it will take a large scale change in our collective professional mind set to implement them widely. Many amongst our own profession still feel there is a stigma attached to an admission of mental ill health. It is this stigma that stops students and doctors seeking the help they need in a timely fashion, and so instead they find themselves trapped in a downward spiral of avoidance, poor decision making, callous thinking, loss of job satisfaction, and unhappiness. Late intervention means that doctors may already have suffered significant damage to their mental health, to their careers, and to their personal lives by the time they get the help they need. It is for this reason that we see doctors and students walking away from their vocation rather than being rehabilitated back into it. It is the stigma still attached to these issues that stops us taking the advice that we would readily give to our patients.

Accepting that burnout is something that almost all doctors will experience to some degree at some point in their career feels like a negative message but, in fact, recognising that this is the case lies at the heart of making jobs within medicine more rewarding, satisfying, and ultimately of better service to our patients.

By engaging with the institutions that govern our profession, by seeking ways to diversify our careers through research, through entrepreneurship, or by embracing different roles within our world, and by actively seeking new and more efficient ways to work, we can improve our own working lives and, perhaps more importantly, the systems within which we work.

The current climate of low morale and rising levels of burnout might not seem like fertile ground in which to grow a brighter future for ourselves and our colleagues, but dissatisfaction can be a powerful driver for change. Now, then, is the time to take advantage of this widespread dissatisfaction and instigate this much-needed change.

REFERENCES

1. The Physicians Foundation. 2012. Survey of America's Physicians.
2. Royal College of Anaesthetists. 2017. Morale and Welfare Survey.
3. Staten & Lawson (eds). 2017. *Combatting Burnout in General Practice*. London: CRC Press.

Index

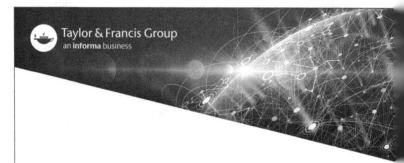

Printed in the United States
by Baker & Taylor Publisher Services